Self-Management of Depression

Daniel P. marshall MD

323-1200

Self-Management of Depression

A Manual for Mental Health and
Primary Care Professionals

Albert Yeung

Greg Feldman

Maurizio Fava

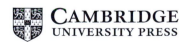

CAMBRIDGE UNIVERSITY PRESS
Cambridge, New York, Melbourne, Madrid, Cape Town, Singapore, São Paulo, Delhi

Cambridge University Press
The Edinburgh Building, Cambridge CB2 8RU, UK

Published in the United States of America by Cambridge University Press, New York

www.cambridge.org
Information on this title: www.cambridge.org/9780521710084

First published 2010

Printed in the United Kingdom at the University Press, Cambridge

A catalogue record for this publication is available from the British Library

Library of Congress Cataloguing in Publication data
Yeung, Albert, 1955–
Self-management of depression : a manual for mental health and primary care professionals /
Albert Yeung, Gregory Feldman, Maurizio Fava.
  p.   ;   cm.
Includes bibliographical references and index.
ISBN 978-0-521-71008-4 (hardcover)
1. Depression, Mental – Treatment.   2. Self-care, Health.   I. Feldman, Gregory.   II. Fava, M.
(Maurizio)   III. Title.
[DNLM: 1. Depressive Disorder – therapy.   2. Patient Participation.   3. Psychotherapy –
methods.   4. Self Care – methods.   WM 171 Y48s 2010]
RC537.Y48   2010
616.85'2706 – dc22   2009028643

ISBN 978-0-521-71008-4 paperback

To my wife Sharon, and our two daughters, Janet and Alicia, with love.

−AY

I wish to thank my wife, Amy, and our two sons, Benjamin and Samuel, for their support and inspiration.

−GF

I could not do what I do without the extraordinary help and support from my wife Stefania and our son Giovanni.

−MF

Contents

Absolutly no info and

diet, alcohol, Nutritional Support
  or Nondrug Rx~ ie SAME
    1- Tryptoplan
No section on "light" Therpy
    (ie SAD's Nights)

Preface

From the clinician's perspective, a key component of self-management of depression is connecting patients with enduring resources to monitor and manage their symptoms. As such, throughout this book, we provide patient hand-outs containing information to guide their use of self-management, including tips for initiating and sustaining an exercise program and selecting a peer support group, as well as lists of links to Internet resources where patients can find self-assessment tools, information about learning meditation, and web-based cognitive behavioral therapy programs. These hand-outs may be photocopied and distributed by the purchaser of this book to patients. These hand-outs are also available for download at no cost at http://www.cambridge.org/9780521710084.

Acknowledgments

We would like to acknowledge our outstanding colleagues in the Depression Clinical and Research Program at Massachusetts General Hospital for their early brainstorming with us about this book when it was in its infancy. In addition, we are grateful for the expert consultation provided by the following colleagues at various stages of this book's development: Jim Cartreine, Ph.D., at Harvard Medical School and the Beth Israel Deaconess Medical Center; Richard Bedrosian, Ph.D., of MySelfHelp.com in Northboro, MA; Dennis Tannenbaum, M.D., at Sentiens in Perth, Australia; Barbara Gentile, Ph.D., at Simmons College; and Sheri Johnson, Ph.D., at University of California–Berkeley. We would also like to thank Katie James and Richard Marley at Cambridge University Press for their support and knowledgeable assistance with this project at all stages of its development. We greatly appreciate the following research assistants who provided invaluable assistance with the preparation of this manuscript: Molly Kerrigan, Caitlin Novero, Hillary Forbes, and Laurie Low at Simmons College; and Lily Zhong and Vicky Lepoutre at the Benson Henry Institute for Mind Body Medicine at Massachusetts General Hospital.

In addition, I (GF) would like to acknowledge that my work on this project was supported in part by a grant from the President's Fund for Faculty Excellence at Simmons College.

The use of self-management for depression

Major depressive disorder – commonly referred to as "depression" – is a prevalent, debilitating, costly, often chronic, and potentially fatal condition. As many as 17% of people will experience major depressive disorder (MDD) in their lifetime (American Psychiatric Association [APA], 2000). The World Health Organization (2001) predicts that depression will become the second largest cause of disability worldwide by 2020. The economic burden of depression in the United States is estimated to be over $83 billion per year, including direct medical costs, workplace costs, and suicide-related mortality costs (Greenberg et al., 2003). Despite its high prevalence, many individuals with depression have difficulty accessing adequate care (Kessler et al., 2003; Hirshfeld et al., 1997). In the United States and abroad, there are shortages of trained mental health professionals to address the increasing prevalence of depression. New strategies are needed for delivering efficient and effective treatment for depression. Self-management holds promise as a strategy for identifying, treating, and managing depression.

What is self-management?

Self-management can be defined as the methods, skills, and strategies by which individuals effectively direct their own activities toward the achievement of specific objectives. It usually includes goal-setting, planning, scheduling, task tracking, self-evaluation, self-intervention, and self-development. In health care, self-management typically refers to the training, skill acquisition, and interventions through which patients who suffer from a disease or a chronic condition may take care of themselves and manage their illnesses.

Why is self-management relevant for depression?

The principles of self-management have been successfully implemented in managing many chronic illnesses, including diabetes, congestive heart disease, and obesity. Self-management involves a collaborative relationship between the patient and one or more primary care or mental health clinicians. The patient is taught and encouraged to (1) view treatment as a collaborative process, (2) actively self-monitor symptoms, and (3) supplement professionally delivered interventions (antidepressant medication and psychotherapy) by using evidence-based, self-administered interventions; for instance, structured physical exercise programs and interactive computer programs that teach effective coping strategies. Self-management has the potential to empower individuals already receiving treatment and provide them with additional resources. It can also increase access to treatment for individuals in geographically remote areas. By shifting more responsibility for symptom management to the patient, a greater number of patients may access treatment, the efficacy of standard therapies may be enhanced, risk of relapse may potentially be decreased, and clinician time may be reduced, thus freeing up clinicians to treat additional patients. Finally, self-management has the potential to reduce costs associated with untreated or poorly managed depression, including health care expenses, disability, and lost workplace productivity.

Overview of this chapter

As previously mentioned, the principles of self-management have been successfully implemented in managing many chronic illnesses. In this chapter, we will present principles and theoretical models describing approaches to management of chronic illness based upon reviews of programs or treatments found to be successful in managing chronic illness through self-management. We will explain how a collaborative clinician–patient relationship is used to empower patients and how this can be contrasted with traditional approaches to health education. Next, we will preview the approaches to self-management for depression that will be discussed in greater detail in later chapters. From there, we will discuss why patients' own attempts at self-management of depression may be unsuccessful. Finally, we will conclude by discussing six essential components of self-management and discussing research support for collaborative care and self-management in treating several chronic illnesses, including depression.

A note on how to read this book

The overall goal of this book is to provide primary care physicians and nurses, psychiatrists, psychologists, social workers, and other professional caregivers with the knowledge and tools for making their work with patients with depression more efficient and effective by integrating self-management treatment strategies with conventional professionally delivered treatment modalities.

Consistent with the collaborative nature of self-management, this book will not present a prescription of a rigid sequence of actions a clinician must take in order to truly use self-management in his/her practice. This book contains no "one-size-fits all" recommendations. Instead, our goal is to present information about approaches used across multiple studies that have worked to increase collaborative care and self-management. Readers are encouraged to think about their own clinical setting and the needs of the patients they serve in deciding how to apply the models and interventions described.

Who needs self-management?

If we use a broad definition of self-management, it can be argued that everyone needs and performs some form of self-management. Every day, we are faced with stress and challenges in life that frequently lead to distress and emotional problems. To maintain a sense of well-being, people usually have their own ways to obtain a sense of emotional well-being. When people suffer from an illness, they may need specific knowledge or skills to respond so that they can recover from the illness, avoid its worsening, or prevent recurrences. There is extensive literature on how environmental factors, emotions, and lifestyles affect health. We make decisions every day on the type of food we eat, how often and how much we eat, how much physical exercise we do, how much time we spend working and resting, the type of activities we do for recreation, the people with whom we interact, and the way in which we interact with them. All of these can be considered as some forms of self-management. We know that what we eat affects our body chemistry. A diet rich in saturated fat could increase our blood cholesterol; elevated cholesterol level is a known risk factor for atherosclerosis, heart disease, and stroke; high caloric intake may lead to becoming overweight and obese; and consuming too many sweets and carbohydrates among people who are predisposed to diabetes may lead to elevated levels of blood glucose.

Patients with chronic medical conditions, in particular, live with and self-manage their illnesses continuously. Each day, they decide what they eat, whether they will exercise, and in some conditions like diabetes and asthma, the dosages of medications to use. For successful management of their diseases, it is important that patients have an in-depth understanding of their illnesses so that they are able to meticulously monitor their symptoms, adopt healthy lifestyles, and implement treatment plans for their illnesses. Depression can be considered a recurrent and/or chronic disorder in that episodes of depression may recur and/or last for many years. Furthermore, even for patients who recover from an episode, the majority will relapse (APA, 2000). In fact, at least 60% of patients with one episode of depression will experience a second. Seventy percent of those with two episodes experience a third, and 90% of those with three episodes will have a fourth. This book explores what people can do to manage their symptoms of depression through behavioral change, such as lifestyle modification, and how health care providers can encourage and guide patients' use of these self-management strategies.

Self-management of chronic medical conditions

Epidemiology of chronic disease

The population of the United States has a demographic profile that is rapidly aging. As a result, the prevalence of chronic medical conditions associated with aging is increasing at a fast pace. Today, chronic disease is the main reason why people in the United States seek health care, and they consume 70% or more of health care spending (Holman & Lorig, 2000). In most industrialized nations and in many developing countries, chronic diseases are the main causes of disability and death. According to data published by the World Bank, 5 of the 10 leading causes of burdens of diseases (projected years living in disability due to the condition) were chronic diseases, including ischemic heart disease, cerebrovascular disease, HIV/AIDS, unipolar depression, and chronic obstructive pulmonary disease (Lopez et al., 2006).

Goals of treating chronic diseases

The goals in the treatment of chronic disease are very different from those in the treatment of acute illnesses. For acute diseases, the goal of treatment is to eradicate the causes of the disease so that the patients can return to normal. Chronic diseases are irreversible or relapsing conditions that are either persistent or run a wax-and-wane course. They typically interact with environmental factors, recur and remit throughout the lives of the patients, and tend to require continuous and complex management. The goal of chronic diseases treatment is not cure, but to support patients in managing their own diseases so that they can maintain satisfying, pleasurable, and independent lifestyles. There is increasing evidence that self-management educational and supportive interventions are effective in helping patients with chronic diseases change their risky behaviors or become better self-managers, and in improving outcomes across a range of chronic illnesses.

Management of chronic illnesses: is the current US health care system adequate?

With the rising prevalence of chronic illnesses and the increasing attention they have received in recent years, effective treatment has been devised for many of the chronic diseases, such as hypertension, depression, diabetes, and asthma. Yet, less than half of patients with hypertension, depression, diabetes, and asthma are receiving appropriate treatment, according to a recent Institute of Medicine report (Wagner et al., 2001a). This lack of adequate care was partly attributed to the high demands on medical care due to the rapid increase in the prevalence of chronic diseases and partly to the US health care system, which was designed to manage acute illnesses or injuries and not chronic diseases. "The focus of the current health care system is on the immediate problem, its rapid recognition and exclusion of more serious alternative diagnoses, and the initiation of professional treatment. Under such a system, the patient's role was largely passive" (Wagner et al., 2001a).

The current primary care health delivery system provides little support to handle the needed lifestyle changes, such as changes in diet, exercise, and stress management, required by people with chronic medical conditions. It also does not provide patients with assistance in creating and maintaining new meaningful life-roles regarding jobs, family, and friends, nor does it provide guidance in ways to cope with the anger, fear, frustration, and sadness that can be part of the experience of a chronic condition. People with chronic conditions have to successfully overcome all these challenges before they can effectively manage their chronic conditions (Corbin & Strauss, 1988). Wagner (2000) concluded that there was a need to redesign the current health care delivery system in order to provide better care to patients with chronic medical conditions and diseases.

The Chronic Care Model

To improve care for chronic disease, Wagner studied successful quality improvement programs for many chronic diseases, including diabetes, congestive heart failure, asthma, hyperlipidemia, and depression. Wagner (1998) found that what these successful programs had in common was that they used a multifaceted approach and all included one or more of the following provider-oriented components: continuing education to physicians, organizational changes in personnel to facilitate patients' visits and follow-up, information systems changes, and patient-oriented interventions. Based on these observations, Wagner (1998) designed the Chronic Care Model for the management of chronic diseases.

The Chronic Care Model typically includes setting up a clinical information system registry, delivery system design, decision support, self-management support, and community resources and policies. The development of computerized disease registries facilitates systematic tracking of patients with a specific condition, sending reminders to patients regarding their follow-up visits to avoid delayed treatment, monitoring treatment outcomes, and providing feedback to practitioners. The designing of the delivery system involves defining roles in the patient treatment team to delegate responsibilities among the multidisciplinary team members. The goal is to ensure continuity of care by the treatment team and to ensure regular follow-up. Decision support involves the development and implementation of evidence-based guidelines using provider education, reminders, and increased interactions among generalists and specialists.

Of particular relevance to this book, self-management support is considered a key element in the Chronic Care Model. Self-management support emphasizes the patients' central role in managing their illness and provides effective behavior change interventions and ongoing support with peers or professionals. Establishment of community resources and policies involves setting up partnerships with community organizations to develop evidence-based programs and identifying effective programs in the community in which patients may participate. The Chronic Care Model has been found to be successful in over 300 diverse health care systems in the context of quality-improvement efforts for asthma, congestive heart failure, depression, diabetes, prevention of frailty in the elderly, and provision of an extremely helpful organizing framework for these diverse quality improvement efforts (Wagner et al., 2001b; Glasgow et al., 2001).

In the Chronic Care Model, optimal chronic care is achieved when a prepared, proactive practice team interacts with an informed, activated patient. It embraces two major components: collaborative care and self-management education. Collaborative care is established on a new form of patient-physician relationship in which physicians and patients form a partnership relationship. Together, they make health care decisions and implement the treatment plan. In the following sections, we will discuss the principles of self-management with a focus on how the collaborative clinician–patient relationship can promote self-management.

The principles of self-management

In this section, we describe some of the key principles for self-management, including the importance of empowering patients and promoting their self-efficacy through the use of collaborative care and self-management education.

Empowering patients through shared decision making

To live the best quality of life, patients with chronic conditions need to be expert in managing their own conditions and to understand how to avoid intensifying or having relapses of their conditions. Patients are no longer passive recipients of medical care. They need to be partners in the process and to play a key role in making decisions about the choice of treatment, interpreting and managing changes in their conditions, coping with emotional reactions, implementing behavioral changes, and utilizing medical and community resources. Empowering patients facilitates the effective and efficient delivery of health care. It has been found that adopting patient's views about their illnesses was associated with higher satisfaction, better treatment adherence, and greater continuity of care (Holman & Lorig, 2000).

Patients who self-manage their chronic medical conditions are given the responsibility to handle their chronic conditions. This parallels the current trend in medicine to include patients as partners in medical decision making. The 1982 President's Commission for the Study of Ethical Problems in Medicine and Biomedicine and Behavioral Research emphasizes the importance of including patients as partners in medical decision making. The Commission's recommendation can be viewed as a continuation of the movement in the past several decades in the United States to increasingly acknowledge patients' autonomy and to provide full information to patients about their illness so that they can make informed decisions about their treatment. Ignoring a patient's right to know about their medical condition and to take part in deciding on their treatment is considered a denial of their autonomy and a violation of current medical ethics.

As successful implementation of self-management of chronic medical condition requires partnership from the patients, this shifts away from the traditional medical model to the shared decision-making model. The traditional medical model is a more paternalistic model in which the doctor determines the best treatment for the patient. The physician provides the patient with select information in order to obtain his/her agreement with the procedure. The shared decision-making model involves both the doctor and the patient sharing information about treatment options in order to arrive at a consensus regarding the preferred treatment options. As Charles and colleagues (1997) state, "Shared decision making is seen as a mechanism for decreasing the informational and power asymmetry between doctors and patients by increasing patients' information, sense of autonomy and/or control over treatment decisions that affect their well-being." Shared decision making addresses a limitation of the traditional medical model that assumes the doctor is the unquestioned expert and unilateral decision maker. In fact, doctors cannot always make the best decision for their patients because they may know little about the individual priorities of their patients or they assess them incorrectly. The advantages to patients of participating in the decision of what problems to tackle is apparent; while professionals know what is most helpful to manage the disease, patients know their priorities and their limitations and what is feasible to implement given their personal and social environment.

It is believed that by taking into consideration the individual's goals and priorities and his/her view regarding the advantages and disadvantages of different options, shared decision making helps patients better understand and self-manage their disorder (Hamann et al., 2003). In addition, shared decision making empowers patients by arousing their internal motivation to take responsibility and manage their own conditions. This is more effective than external motivation from professionals for inducing lifestyle changes.

Promoting patients' self-efficacy through self-management education

The central concept in self-management is to enhance self-efficacy, the belief and confidence that patients can make changes in their lives. Self-efficacy is a concept introduced by Bandura as one core aspect of his social cognitive theory (Bandura, 1997). In the context of self-management, self-efficacy is complementary to the idea of empowerment just discussed. While empowerment encourages patients to feel that they are equal with the clinicians in making decisions about their treatment, self-management training promotes patients' self-efficacy by encouraging and guiding them to carry out behaviors to attain their desired goals. Patients with chronic illnesses rely on themselves, with the help of their health providers, family, friends, worksites, and community resources, to adopt healthy lifestyles and behaviors which are beneficial to successful management of their illnesses. According to Bandura, self-efficacy beliefs determine how people feel, think, and motivate themselves to behave. Person with high perceived self-efficacy believe in their capabilities to produce changes to affect their lives. They tend to conduct a more active and self-determined life course. They set up challenging goals for themselves and maintain strong commitment to the goals. When faced with setbacks, they heighten and sustain their efforts and quickly recover their sense of self-efficacy. They attribute setbacks or failures to insufficient effort or deficient knowledge and skills, which are acquirable. They handle challenges with the confidence that challenges can be overcome. People with such efficacious outlooks tend to produce personal accomplishments, have reduced stress, and are less vulnerable to depression.

In contrast, people with low self-efficacy doubt their capabilities and avoid difficult tasks, which they view as personal threats. They tend to have low aspirations and weak commitment to the goals they choose to pursue. When faced with challenges, their confidence is shaken, they dwell on their personal deficiencies, and they start to worry about the obstacles they will encounter and all the possible adverse outcomes. In the end, they tend to succumb to obstacles and to give up their goals. They find it hard to recover their sense of efficacy following failure or setbacks. They easily fall victim to stress and depression.

Based on the theory of self-efficacy, self-management in clinical care is geared to provide the resources and the training in a systematic manner so that people with chronic medical conditions acquire the skills and the confidence to be self-efficacious in the management of their conditions.

The theory of self-efficacy is based on the theme of individual responsibility, implying that people are responsible for their own behavior (Lorig & Holman,

2003). Under such a theme, patients are encouraged and taught the skills needed to take an active part in the management of their chronic medical conditions. They are discouraged from acting as a passive recipient and waiting for health professionals to take away their problems. From a practical point of view, patients with a chronic disease are the ones who perform their day-to-day management and decide whether to engage in a health-promoting activity, such as exercise or diet control. It is impossible, without compromising patients' autonomy as well as privacy, to constantly supervise patients with chronic diseases over the entire extended course of their illnesses.

Studies have shown that patients who are confident in their ability to manage their illnesses are the ones with the best health outcomes (Schwarzer, 1992). Based on the self-efficacy theory, there are four ways that confidence can be increased. One way is for health professionals to collaborate with patients on setting short-term achievable goals so that patients will master new skills. A second way is for patients to meet someone like themselves so that they can learn disease management through modeling. This can be done through patient groups, peer leaders, and, more recently, chat rooms via the Internet. The third way is to assist patients to understand the multiple causes of their symptoms. In doing so, patients may understand that many of their own behaviors may contribute to their illnesses and that the disease can be better controlled through changes in their lifestyles. The fourth way is social persuasion. Praise and encouragement concerning patient's accomplishments by health professionals, friends, and family are important in increasing patients' confidence in what they can do in the control of their illnesses.

Self-management education is designed to enhance self-efficacy so that patients feel confident in managing challenges in their lives. In traditional patient education, health care professionals define the problems and decide what information and skills to teach. Self-management education allows patients to identify their problems that may or may not be related to the disease. It provides techniques to help patients make decisions and to take appropriate actions to respond to changes in their diseases. While traditional health education pro- vides disease-specific information and technical skills related to the disease, self-management education provides problem-solving skills that are relevant to the consequences of the chronic condition in general. The underlying theory behind traditional patient education is that the health professionals know the answers and what is the best for the patient. Once the patient acquires the knowledge, they will be able to implement it and produce better clinical out- comes. Self-management education theorizes that greater patient confidence in his/her capacity to make life-improving changes yields better clinical outcomes (Bodenheimer et al., 2002).

A central feature of self-management education involves patients asking to generate their short-term action plans based on what they want to do. The purpose of action plans is to fuel the patients' internal motivation and to give patients confidence in managing their disease. It has been shown that patients who actually make action plans have better outcomes (Bodenheimer et al., 2002).

Traditional patient education in the clinic is usually provided by a health care professional. For self-management education, a health professional, a peer leader, or another patient can be the educator, and it often happens in a group format. The use of lay resources and group settings in self-management education increases the access of self-management education to patients with chronic diseases in an economical and efficient way.

Self-management of depression

The concept of clinical depression

Clinicians who treat patients with depression need to know how severe their depression is and whether intervention is warranted. It begs the fundamental question: "When does depression become a clinical condition and a disease?" "In the human population, is there a natural or continuous distribution of depressive symptoms and we simply consider people clinically depressed if they fall on the more severe side of the continuum, or do we consider clinical depression a distinct disease entity that involves a unique pathological mechanism?"

Instead of directly answering these questions, the American Psychiatric Association (2000) adopts an atheoretical approach in the *Diagnostic and Statistical Manual Fourth Edition Text Revision* (DSM-IV-TR) and defines depressive disorders based on the presence of a cluster of symptoms, duration of symptoms, and whether they have caused significant distress or functional impairment to the person suffering from the symptoms. Using major depressive disorder (MDD) as the example, its diagnosis involves the presence of five of more of the depressive symptoms, one of which needs to be depressed mood or loss of interest or pleasure in the activities that used to be enjoyable. Other symptoms in the DSM-IV-TR diagnostic criteria for MDD include changes in sleep or eating patterns, agitation or retardation, fatigue, inability to concentrate, indecisiveness, feelings of worthlessness or excessive guilt, and suicidal thoughts. The symptoms would need to last for 2 weeks or more, and must have caused either significant subject distress or impairment in social and occupational functioning. In addition to these symptoms described in the DSM-IV-TR diagnostic criteria, depressed patients may also demonstrate symptoms associated with depression, including anxiety, irritability, preoccupation with physical heath or complaints of pain, brooding, obsessive rumination, and pessimism (APA, 2000).

The DSM-IV-TR criteria of MDD, informed by research and established by expert consensus meetings, offers an agreed-upon definition which has helped increase the reliability of this most commonly diagnosed form of clinical depression. Other less commonly diagnosed depressive disorders in the DSM-IV include minor depressive disorder, dysthymic disorder, and depressive disorder not otherwise specified. Because our understanding of minor depression and dysthymia is significantly less compared with MDD, clinical depression refers to MDD in this book unless it is otherwise specified. The existence of the DSM-IV-TR diagnostic criteria has facilitated considerable progress in extensive clinical studies to provide the evidence for understanding the mechanism of depression as well as for the establishment of treatment guidelines for depressive disorders.

What causes depression?

While the exact cause of depression is unclear, it has been known for many years that depression tends to run in families. First-degree relatives of individuals with MDD are two to three times more likely to develop the disorder as compared with people in the general population (Klein et al., 2002). Yet, positive family history could be either a genetic factor or an upbringing influence. Carefully conducted studies of twins suggest that both genetic factors and environmental factors play a role in causing depression, with genetic factors accounting for roughly 37% of the variance in who does and does not develop depression (Sullivan et al., 2000). In addition to family history, people who go through stressful events, suffer from chronic medical illnesses, and have cognitive vulnerabilities such as low self-esteem and a negative view of the world also have higher risks of developing depression. An increasingly accepted model is the diathesis-stress model, which suggests that depression is most likely to occur in individuals who have a preexisting genetic or cognitive vulnerability and also experience significant life stress. This model has received support in several recent studies (e.g. Caspi et al., 2003).

Use of self-management for managing clinical depression

While there is abundant literature on the treatment of depressive disorders, there have been much less systematic studies on self-management of depression. There are several important questions about self-management for depression: Is self-management effective for treating MDD, either as a stand-alone therapy or as an adjunct therapy to supplement pharmacotherapy and/or psychotherapy, the conventional therapies for MDD? Can self-management be used to prevent episodes of depression in individuals who are at elevated risk due to family history or stressful life circumstances, including chronic medical illness? Despite the fact that medication treatment has been shown effective for treatment of MDD (Agency for Health Care Policy and Research [AHCPR], 1993), some patients prefer not to take medications due to medical reasons (e.g. during pregnancy), or they may not be able to tolerate side effects of medications. Psychotherapeutic interventions, including cognitive behavioral therapy (CBT) and interpersonal therapy (IPT), have been found to be effective treatments for depression (AHCPR, 1993). Yet, there are not sufficient numbers of well-trained psychotherapists in these psychotherapeutic modalities in the United States. The overall shortage of psychotherapists trained in the treatment of depression is much more dramatic in non-Western countries. For many patients, self-management of depression may be the only treatment available. For people who are receiving pharmacotherapy or psychotherapy, self-management could be a useful adjunctive therapy to the existing treatment. For patients who are at high risk for developing depression or have had previous episodes of depression, self-management could be used as preventive measures to the onset, recurrence, or relapse of depression.

Approaches to self-management of depression

Based on existing evidence, the different chapters in this book discuss how clinicians can help their patients manage depression and promote well-being through self-management. In addition to describing specific self-management strategies, we will focus on how clinicians can work collaboratively with their patients to help them reset priorities in their lives, challenge maladaptive and irrational thinking patterns that may undermine self-care, and discover the motivation to accomplish goals they set for themselves. There is no shortage of information for patients about depression and recommendations for self-management available in the popular press and on the Internet. However, much of this information may be unreliable (Ernst & Schmidt, 2004; Griffiths & Christensen, 2000). In this book, we will clearly explain the state of empirical support for each of the methods described.

Many effective psychological interventions have been developed in the past several decades, and a lot of this knowledge and these skills can be acquired by self-learning, as information is now easily accessible for people who seek it. In Chapter 4, we will review a variety of self-help versions of CBT that can be found in widely available books and interactive computer programs with a focus on programs that have received empirical support through rigorous studies. In Chapter 5, we will review evidence supporting physical exercise as a form of depression self-management to complement more well-known benefits of exercise, such as maintaining body weight, lowering blood cholesterol levels, and strengthening skeletal muscles and our hearts.

The importance of a multidisciplinary approach has been emphasized by Wagner (2000) for treatment of chronic illnesses, including depression. While individuals can obtain much of the knowledge on depression self-help on their own, they also benefit from professional advice from primary care physicians and mental health specialists. Some clinical programs use care managers to coordinate all the care for the patients and to motivate, monitor, and provide support to patients. We will discuss this approach to self-management in Chapter 2.

Many cultures have developed skills to influence the mind through meditation. In recent years, such a practice has been extensively used and studied in the West. We will review different forms of meditation and relaxation practices, the proposed mechanisms of action, and the potential benefits of these practices on depression in Chapter 6. Family interaction, as well as the quality of interpersonal relationships, is known to have tremendous effects on peoples' emotions. In fact, in many collectivistic cultures, peoples' existences and identities are defined by the roles they play in their society. Ideally, family members of people suffering from depression should be involved in the treatment as they frequently suffer the most, living around patients who are afflicted by depression. We discuss the role of family and peers in Chapter 7, which focuses on the role of social support in self-management.

Do people with depression need clinicians to effectively use self-management?

Most people who are in distress or having difficulty functioning start assessing their lifestyles and open themselves to experimenting with new approaches, hoping to get relief from mood symptoms. In other words, they explore some sort of self-management. We would argue that although this process of self-regulation works for many individuals, it typically is impaired for individuals with depression. For instance, when people wait to act until depression symptoms can no longer be ignored, it may be too late, as loss in motivation and energy may impair efforts at coping or self-care. As such, early detection of symptom changes is crucial. Thus in Chapter 3, we describe the role of providing patients with information about depression symptoms and tools for self-assessment to monitor symptom levels.

Self-management measures are usually chosen to address the assumed causes of depression or to promote an overall sense of well-being. Some people try to get more rest if they have been overworked, a common occurrence in today's society. Others try to get rejuvenated by taking a vacation. Many people may start to make changes in their personal habits, such as limiting the number of late-night movies or television shows they watch, if this habit causes day-time fatigue. People with sleep problems may find help from learning how to maintain sleep hygiene. It may sound too simplistic: the use of sleep hygiene measures may be all that is needed for some to overcome their depressive symptoms; those who have difficulty at work may start to make adjustments in their work habits or address interpersonal relationships to improve the environment at work.

Between the common-sense self-help described above and the increasingly available self-assessment tools and evidence-based self-help books and computerized self-treatment programs, the question arises whether clinicians still have a useful role in patients' self-management of depression. Unfortunately, the self-management strategies that individuals with depression discover on their own are not always optimal and may be counterproductive or even dangerous. In fact, some will turn to alcohol, nicotine, or other illegal mood-altering substances. Others may begin avoiding aspects of their life that cause distress. Each of these strategies produces short-term relief, but is potentially costly in the long term. Furthermore, as noted previously, without the assistance of an informed clinician, patients may seek out self-help programs promoted in the popular media that have little or no research supporting their efficacy. From our own study on recent immigrants in Boston, most of them had explored different forms of self-management and alternative treatments for their depression for years before seeking professional help from mental health providers (Yeung & Kam, 2005). The fact that the patients in our study eventually sought treatment suggests that self-identified self-management strategies may only be partially or temporarily effective at best. Based on learning theories, we will discuss the importance of health professionals in guiding, motivating, and changing the behaviors of patients in their efforts to take care of their depression in Chapter 2.

The key resources and support for self-management

In 2002, the Robert Wood Johnson Foundation launched the Diabetes Initiative, a national program to both demonstrate and evaluate diabetes self-management promotion in 14 primary care and community settings. The initiative identified several key resources and supports that are needed for successful self-management of diabetes as well as other chronic medical conditions. These key elements are individualized assessment, collaborative goal-setting, skills enhancement, follow-up and support, access to resources in daily life, and continuity of quality clinical care (Fisher et al., 2005).

Individualized assessment

Studies in cross-cultural psychiatry have shown that people from different cultural backgrounds often have very different explanatory models of illness; this refers to the way they understand the nature of the illness, its consequences, and how best to treat it. Arthur Kleinman, a Harvard anthropologist, studied depression in China in the 1970s and found that Chinese patients with depression rarely reported depressed mood and that they complained mainly of somatic symptoms (Kleinman, 1982). He concluded that depression is not the "idiom" of language to communicate distress for Chinese populations, which is the result of psychological and sociocultural factors. The authors of this book have recently investigated the illness beliefs of underserved immigrants in Boston who were diagnosed with MDD and found that many of them were not familiar with depression, a concept that originated in the West. Most of them did not recognize that they had a treatable illness, or many attributed their symptoms to their existing medical conditions.

To successfully engage individuals with diverse personal views of their illness, seasoned health professionals need to learn to share the individuals' viewpoints and put things in their cultural context. To be able to tailor to each individual, it is helpful to understand patients' concepts of illness, ideas of medical treatment, expectations on treatment outcomes, and worries about possible side effects from treatment and long-term effects from the illness.

The recent trend in medicine has focused on understanding the biological mechanisms of diseases. Yet, for the person with the disease, it is a very personal experience which needs to be incorporated into the different psychosocial aspects of his/her life. To obtain an example from a clinician working with a client on self-management interventions for hypertension and diabetes, a clinician expressed concern about the fluctuations of blood pressure and the meticulous control of blood sugar to a patient and asked the patient why he was not taking the medications as prescribed. The patient informed the physician that he had lost his home during a recent hurricane and his focus then was how to find a job and having a safe environment to live in. Similarly, many patients juggle marital issues, financial difficulties, and other medical and psychosocial issues in their lives. To the patient, these psychosocial issues are frequently considered more urgent than the disease itself.

Health professionals need to keep in mind that their medical training offers them a framework to understand the disease, which needs to fit into the illness beliefs and the priorities in the lives of the patients, who are ultimately the consumers of medical services. We will discuss this concept of individualized assessment in Chapter 3, Self-assessment instruments for depression.

Collaborative goal-setting

The aim of collaborative goal-setting is to empower patients and emphasize that they have authority over the management of their illness. Patients are explicitly informed that they can participate in deciding on treatment choices and that they share the responsibility in the success of their treatment. Collaborative goal-setting takes away the managerial role of health professionals. By increasing the patient's sense of ownership of the problem and personal stake in treatment, adherence to treatment can be expected to increase (Anderson & Funnell, 2000).

There are numerous approaches to collaborative goal-setting. Motivational interviewing is one popular approach which originated from treatment for people who are dependent on alcohol and drugs and has been applied to other populations. Motivational interviewing was developed by Miller and Rollnick (2002), and it accepts the fact that patients may be at different levels of readiness to change their behavior at question. It is based upon four principles: (1) express empathy to patients' perspectives, (2) point out the discrepancy between how clients want their lives to be versus how they currently are, (3) accept patients who continue to be resistant to change, and (4) encourage patients' autonomy and confidence. Motivational interviewing uses a non-judgmental and non-confrontational approach and attempts to increase client's awareness of the potential problem causes, consequences experienced, and risks faced as a result of the behavior in question. Therapists have found motivational interviewing useful to help clients suffering from different health and medical conditions to envision a better future and become motivated to achieve it by recognizing that they have authority over their illnesses.

Skills enhancement

Skills that are important for successful self-management include self-monitoring, challenging negative and unproductive thinking, problem solving, and resisting the temptation of maladaptive behavior patterns. Along with eating a healthy diet and staying physically active to enhance a healthy lifestyle in general, these skills are applicable to a wide variety of chronic conditions.

In contrast to conventional approaches to health education that tend to provide only didactic lectures, the self-management approach focuses on improving individual skills and their successful application in daily life. Self-management education is usually delivered through multiple meetings, often in group format to introduce and rehearse skills, and people are encouraged to test out these skills in the real world between meetings. The five-step approach of the Problem Solving Therapy (D'Zurilla & Nezu, 1999) has been found to be very useful in teaching problem-solving skills. These five steps are as follows:

(1) Attitude. Before attempting to solve the problem, individuals adopt a positive, optimistic attitude toward the problem and their problem-solving ability.

(2) Define. The individuals define the problem by obtaining relevant facts, identifying obstacles that inhibit goal achievement, and specifying a realistic goal.

(3) Alternatives. Based upon a well-defined problem, persons are directed to next generate a variety of different alternatives for overcoming the identified obstacles and achieving the problem-solving goal.

(4) Predict. After generating a list of alternatives, people are directed to predict both the positive and negative consequences of each alternative in order to choose the one that has the highest probability of achieving the problem-solving goal, while additionally minimizing costs and maximizing benefits.

(5) Try-out. The chosen solutions are tried out in real life and their effects are monitored.

If people with chronic medical conditions are satisfied with the results, the problem is solved and they should engage in self-reinforcement. If they are not satisfied, they are then directed to go back to the first step and try again in order to find a more effective solution. This technique was originally developed as a behavioral treatment for depression, but has subsequently been applied with success to a wide range of challenges, such as management of diabetes and cancer, and for managing psychosocial problems and negative moods, such as hostility, anger, stress, and anxiety, which are associated with poor health (deGroot et al., 2001; Williams et al., 2003).

Follow-up and support

Norris and colleagues (2001) performed a meta-analysis of self-management programs in diabetes and found improvement in glycemic control in the short term, but the results dropped after 12 months. Research on self-management of diabetes, smoking cessation, and interventions in other areas of health promotion have provided support on the importance of ongoing follow-up and support for behavior change. Because chronic disease management is expected to be needed over the course of the lifetime, it can be argued that patients may benefit from follow-up and support for a long period of time.

We should then pose the question: What kind of support would be necessary during follow-up? Fisher et al. (2005) proposed that follow-up may include continued assistance in refining problem-solving plans and skills, encouragement, and help in responding to new problems. While these are helpful guidelines, more planning and thoughts are needed in order for these guidelines to be implemented.

Follow-up and support may be provided through different forms of communications, including telephone calls, emails, or automated telephone monitoring of patients combined with nurse follow-up, which has been used in the management of diabetes. Telephone counseling has been shown to be effective for the management of diabetes, smoking cessation, and depression (Wasson et al., 1992; Simon et al., 2004).

The use of community-based activities and non-professionals – such as community health workers, lay health workers, health promoters, and health coaches – to provide follow-up and support has grown in popularity. The use of non-professionals and lay workers has the advantage of easy access and less cost. In addition, many patients like the cooperative spirit from peer support more than the authoritative roles of health professionals. Internet-based chat rooms have evolved to become a popular forum for peer support. For instance, clinicians at the Joslin Diabetes Clinic in Boston developed a moderated web-based message board for patients with diabetes, and this program was found to be helpful by the majority of users (Zrebiec, 2005). Patients share their experience, exchange information, and provide mutual support online. With its convenience and low-cost communication, the use of online chat rooms for follow-up support is likely to continue to increase. An old tradition of follow-up and support which has shown renewed interest is the group medical visit, in which patients with a particular condition are scheduled for a 2- to 3-hour group visit. During these visits, patients obtain educational and supportive discussions in addition to their medical assessment.

While the concept of follow-up and support sounds appealing, many questions remain regarding whether every individual with a chronic condition needs or desires it. In the Diabetes Initiative, most patients with diabetes did not present to the monthly support groups (Banister et al., 2004). More work is needed to find out how to provide effective support for each specific condition, who would benefit from it, how to tailor it to the individuals, whether such supports are effective, and lastly, who will pay for it.

Access to resources in daily life

In order to have successful self-management, it is important to have access to resources. For example, the availability of healthy foods is important to having a healthy diet, and having access to safe and appealing facilities increases the motivation for physical activities. A growing body of literature has shown that the "neighborhood environment" has important effects on behavior and health. A recent study in a diverse North Carolina population showed that having walking trails, streetlights, and access to places for physical activities were positively associated with successful engagement of recommended physical activities (Houston et al., 2003).

In another study, it was shown that in the absence of a walkable neighborhood, a phenomenon resulting from unplanned and uncontrolled spreading of urban development, residents walk less during leisure time, weigh more, and have a greater prevalence of hypertension (Ewing et al., 2003). Kahn et al. (2002) performed a systematic review of the effectiveness of various interventions for increasing physical activities and concluded that the creation of or enhanced access to places for physical activity combined with informational outreach activities, school-based physical education, social support in community settings, and individually adapted health behavior change were effective in promoting physical activity.

Continuity of quality clinical care

Self-management and clinical care are complementary components for adequate care of chronic illnesses. Clinical care provides the evidence-based diagnosis, delineates the severity and staging of an illness, and recommends the scope of the treatment according to established treatment guidelines for a specific illness, including the use of medical and surgical interventions, if necessary. Self-management adds the compatible lifestyle, diet, exercise, and behavioral change to maximize the benefits of clinical care and to attain the highest level of functioning possible while living with the illness.

Effectiveness of self-management of chronic illnesses

Self-management of diabetes

A lot has been written on educating and training patients with type 2 diabetes. Yet, the training typically provides traditional education on diabetic information and technical skills, rather than problem-solving skills to develop one's own action plans. The paucity of the use of self-management education hampers the evaluation of its effectiveness with respect to the treatment of diabetes. In 2002, Norris and colleagues (2002) performed a meta-analysis study of the effect on self-management education for glycemic control for adults with type 2 diabetes. They concluded that patient education by itself is not sufficient to improve clinical outcomes, greater patient knowledge is not correlated with improved glycemic control, and education interventions that involve patient collaboration may be more effective than didactic interventions in improving glycemic control. They recommended that self-management interventions for patients with diabetes should include weight management, physical activity, medication management, and blood sugar monitoring.

Self-management of asthma

Asthma is another prevalent chronic condition that requires constant management. A meta-analysis performed in 2001 concluded that patient education alone does not improve health outcomes in adults with asthma (Gibson et al., 2001a). The authors added more current studies and came up with a recent update (Gibson et al., 2001b); they concluded that asthma self-management which involves self-monitoring of peak expiratory flow or of asthma symptoms, coupled with regular medical review and a written action plan, improves health outcomes for adults with asthma.

Bodenheimer et al. (2002) reviewed 23 studies on self-management of asthma which used reasonable control groups. Among these 23 studies measuring outcomes, 11 demonstrated improvements in asthma symptoms; only one study found improvement in measured lung function. They found that studies with self-management action plans had a greater tendency to improve outcomes than those without action plans. In addition, self-management interventions involving mild to moderate asthmatic patients demonstrated a smaller effect than those involving patients with severe asthma.

One of the reviewed studies provided a 5-year follow-up on patients who received self-management education for 1 year. They found that the intervention had led to significant improvement in outcomes in 1 year, but the improvement was not sustained at 5 years (Kaupinnen et al., 2001). This finding raises important questions about how to support patients in continuing to apply effective self-management in an ongoing manner.

Self-management of depression

Similar to treatment of diabetes, studies on the effectiveness of self-management for depression are usually performed in the context of a comprehensive disease management program, making it harder to evaluate the "stand-alone" effects of self-management education. In the UK, there is significant interest on providing self-help for patients with anxiety and depression due to the lack of trained therapists to meet the demand. Consequently, depression management programs (DMPs) have been developed in the UK that involve the use of evidence-based practice guidelines, patient self-management education, provider education, depression screening, routine reporting, and feedback loops between primary care physicians and different health professionals.

Neumeyer-Gromen et al. (2004) performed a systematic review of studies on DMPs for depression and concluded that DMPs enhanced the quality of care of depression. In addition, patient satisfaction and adherence to the treatment regimen improved significantly. The costs involved were within the range of other widely accepted public health improvement programs.

Similarly, Gilbody et al. (2006) reviewed the studies on collaborative care for depression to augment primary care, with features similar to DMPs described above, and concluded that collaborative care is more effective than standard care in improving depression outcomes in short and longer terms.

Conclusion

With the increasing prevalence in chronic medical conditions, self-management will play an ever-increasing role in medical care for prevention, treatment, and rehabilitation of these conditions. To encourage self-management, practitioners need to change from their traditional authoritative role to form partnerships with their patients, who are responsible for modifying their lifestyles to promote health. More studies will be needed to explore how to provide cost-effective self-management education to patients with specific medical conditions, to whom and for how long to provide continued follow-up and support, and how best to involve resources in the community, including non-health professionals, as part of social support for self-management. Self-management of depression remains a work in progress. However, we feel that there is sufficient need, rationale, and evidence of promise that it is time that clinicians consider self-management as an important component of their work with patients who have depression. In the following chapters, we will offer practical suggestions for how to begin.

REFERENCES

Agency for Health Care Policy and Research. Depression Guideline Panel Research: Depression in primary care (vol 2): Treatment of Major Depression. Clinical Practice Guideline, No. 5. Rockville, MD. US Department of Health and Human Services, Public Health Service, Agency for Health Care Policy and Research, 1993.

American Psychiatric Association. *Diagnostic and Statistical Manual of Mental Disorders.* 4th edn, text revision. Washington, DC: American Psychiatric Association; 2000.

Anderson RM, Funnell MM. Compliance and adherence are dysfunctional concepts in diabetes care. *Diabetes Educ.* 2000; 26:597–604.

Bandura A. *Self-Efficacy: The Exercise of Control.* New York, NY: W.H. Freeman; 1997.

Banister NA, Jastrow ST, Hodges V, Loop R, Gillham MB. Diabetes self-management training program in a community clinic improves patient outcomes at modest cost. *J Am Diet Assoc.* 2004; 104:807–810.

Bodenheimer T, Lorig K, Holman H, Grumback K. Patient self-management of chronic disease in primary care. *JAMA.* 2002; 288(19):2469–2475.

Caspi A, Sugden K, Moffitt TE, Taylor A, Craig IW, Harrington H, McClay J, Mill J, Martin J, Braithwaite A, Poulton R. Influence of life stress on depression: moderation by a polymorphism in the 5-HTT gene. *Science.* 2003; 301(5631):386–389.

Charles C, Gafni A, Whelan T. Shred decision-making in the medical encounter: What does it mean? (or it takes at least two to tango). *Soc Sci Med.* 1997; 44(5):681–692.

Corbin J, Strauss A. *Unending Work and Care: Managing Chronic Illness at Home.* San Francisco, CA: Jossey-Bass Publishers; 1988.

deGroot M, Anderson R, Freedland KE, Clouse RE, Lustman PJ. Association of depression and diabetes complications: a meta-analysis. *Psychosom Med.* 2001; 63:619–630.

Depression Initiative. A national program of the Robert Wood Johnson Foundation. Available at http://diabetesnpo.im.wustle.edu. Accessed June 10, 2005.

D'Zurilla TJ, Nezu AM. *Problem-Solving Therapy.* 2nd edn. New York, NY: Springer; 1999.

Ernst E, Schmidt K. Alternative cures for depression: how safe are web sites? *Psychiatry Res.* 2004; 129(3):297–301.

Ewing R, Schmid T, Killingsworth R, Zlot A, Raudenbush S. Relationship between urban sprawl and physical activity, obesity, and morbidity. *Am J Health Promot.* 2003; 18:47–57.

Fisher EB, Brownson CA, O'Toole ML, Shetty G, Anwuri V, Glasgow R. Ecological approaches to self-management: The case of diabetes. *Am J Public Health.* 2005; 95:1523–1535.

Gibson PG, Coughlan J, Wilson AJ, et al. Self-management education and regular practitioner review for adults with asthma [Cochrane Review on CD-ROM]. Oxford, England: Cochrane Library, Update Software; 2001a:[issue 1].

Gibson PG, Coughlan J, Wilson AJ, et al. Limited (information only) asthma education on health outcomes of adults with asthma [Cochrane Review on CD-ROM]. Oxford, England: Cochrane Library, Update Software; 2001b:[issue 4].

Gilbody S, Bower P, Fletcher J, Richards D, Sutton AJ. Collaborative care for depression: a cumulative meta-analysis and review of longer-term outcomes. *Arch Intern Med.* 2006; 27; 166(21):2314–2321.

Glasgow RE, Orleans CT, Wagner EH, Curry SJ, Solberg LI. Does the Chronic Care Model serve also as a template for improving prevention? *Milbank Q.* 2001; 79(4):579–612.

Greenberg PE, Leong SA, Birnbaum HG, Robinson RL. The economic burden of depression with painful symptoms. *J Clin Psychiatry.* 2003; 64(Suppl 7):17–23.

Griffiths KM, Christensen H. Quality of web based information on treatment of depression: cross sectional survey. *BMJ.* 2000; 321(7275):1511–1515.

Hamann J, Leucht S, Kissling W. Shared decision making in psychiatry. *Acta Psychiatr Scand.* 2003; 107(6):403–409.

Hirschfeld RM, Keller MB, Panico S, Arons BS, Barlow D, Davidoff F, Endicott J, Froom J, Goldstein M, Gorman JM, Marek RG, Maurer TA, Meyer R, Phillips K, Ross J, Schwenk TL, Sharfstein SS, Thase ME, Wyatt RJ. The National Depressive and Manic-Depressive Association consensus statement on the undertreatment of depression. *JAMA.* 1997; 277(4):333–340.

Holman H, Lorig K. Patients as partners in managing chronic disease: partnership is a prerequisite for effective and efficient health care. *BMJ.* 2000; 320:526–527.

Houston SL, Evenson KR, Bors P, Gizlice Z. Neighborhood environment, access to places for activity, and leisure-time physical activity in a diverse North Carolina population. *Am J Health Promot.* 2003; 18:58–69.

Kahn EB, Ramsey LT, Brownson RC, Heath GW, Howze EH, Powell KE, Stone EJ, Rajab MW, Corso P. The effectiveness of interventions to increase physical activity: a systematic review. *Am J Prev Med.* 2002; 22:73–107.

Kaupinnen R, Vilkka V, Sintonen H, Klaukka T, Tukiainen H. Long-term economic evaluation of intensive patient education during the first treatment year in newly diagnosed adult asthma. *Respir Med.* 2001; 95:56–63.

Kessler RC, Berglund P, Demler O, Jin R, Koretz D, Merikangas KR, Rush AJ, Walters EE, Wang PS; National Comorbidity Survey Replication. The epidemiology of major depressive disorder: results from the National Comorbidity Survey Replication (NCS-R). *JAMA.* 2003; 289:3095–3105.

Klein DN, Lewinsohn PM, Rohde P, Seeley JR, Durbin CE. Clinical features of major depressive disorder in adolescents and their relatives: impact on familial aggregation, implications for phenotype definition, and specificity of transmission. *J Abnorm Psychol.* 2002; 111(1):98–106.

Kleinman A. Neurasthenia and depression: a study of somatization and culture in China. *Cult Med Psych.* 1982; 6:117–190.

Lopez AD, Mathers CD, Ezzati M, Jamison DT, Murray CJL, eds. *Global Burden of Disease and Risk Factors.* New York, NY: World Bank and Oxford University Press; 2006. Available at http://www.dcp2.org/pubs/GBD/3/Table/3.14

Lorig KR, Holman H. Self-management education: history, definition, outcomes, and mechanisms. *Ann Behav Med.* 2003; 26:1–7.

Miller WR, Rollnick S. *Motivational Interviewing: Preparing People for Change.* 2nd edn. New York, NY: Guilford Press; 2002.

Neumeyer-Gromen A, Lampert T, Stark K, Kallischnigg G. Disease management programs for depression: a systematic review and meta-analysis of randomized controlled trials. *Med Care*. 2004; 42(12):1211–1221.

Norris SL, Engelgau MM, Narayan KM. Effectiveness of self-management training in type 2 diabetes: a systematic review of randomized controlled trials. *Diabetes Care*. 2001; 24:561–587.

Norris SL, Lau J, Smith SJ, Schmid CH, Engelgau M. Self-management education for adults with type 2 diabetes: a meta-analysis of the effect on glycemic control. *Diabetes Care*. 2002; 25:1159–1171.

Schwarzer R, ed. *Self-Efficacy: Thought Control of Action*. Washington, DC: Hemisphere Publishing; 1992.

Simon GE, Ludman EJ, Tutty S, Operskalski B, Von Korff M. Telephone psychotherapy and telephone care management for primary care patients starting antidepressant treatment: a randomized controlled trial. *JAMA*. 2004; 292:935–942.

Sullivan PF, Neale MC, Kendler KS. Genetic epidemiology of major depression: review and meta-analysis. *Am J Psychiatry*. 2000; 157(10):1552–1562.

Wagner EH. Chronic disease management: What will it take to improve care for chronic illness. *Eff Clin Pract*. 1998; 1(1):2–4.

Wagner EH. The role of patient care teams in chronic disease management. *BMJ*. 2000; 320:569–572.

Wagner EH, Austin BT, Davis C, Hindmarsh M, Schaefer J, Bonomi A. Improving chronic illness care: translating evidence into action. *Health Aff (Millwood)*. 2001a; 20(6):64–78.

Wagner EH, Glasgow RE, Davis C, et al. Quality improvement in chronic illness care: a collaborative approach. *Jt Comm J Qual Improv*. 2001b; 27:63–80.

Wasson J, Baudette C, Whaley F, Sauvigne A, Baribeau P, Welch HG. Telephone care as a substitute for routine clinic follow-up. *JAMA*. 1992; 267(13):1788–1793.

Williams RB, Barefoot JC, Schneiderman N. Psychosocial risk factors for cardiovascular disease: more than one culprit at work. *JAMA*. 2003; 290:2190–2192.

World Health Organization. Depression. World Health Organization; 2001. Available at http://www.who.int/mental_health/management/depression/definition/en/

Yeung AS, Kam R. Illness beliefs of depressed Asian Americans in primary care. In Georgiopoulos AM and Rosenbaum JF, eds: *Perspectives in Cross-Cultural Psychiatry*. Philadelphia, PA: Lippincott Williams & Wilkins; 2005, pp 21–36.

Zrebiec JF. Internet communities: do they improve coping with diabetes? *The Diabetes Educ*. 2005; 31(6):825–836.

Care management of depression

Treatment of depression in primary care and the need for a multidisciplinary approach

Recent advances of medical knowledge have enabled greater complexity of treatment regimens for successful treatment of chronic conditions. Many cardiovascular diseases, hypertension, diabetes, and tumors can now be diagnosed relatively early in the process. With effective treatments available, patients with such conditions can be treated successfully. Similarly, recent drug development efforts have provided newer antidepressants and mood stabilizers with improved side effect profiles. With the advent of newer medications and effective psychotherapeutic interventions, most people who suffer from depression can benefit from treatment if symptoms are identified and treated.

It may not be apparent why primary care clinics are important for the treatment of depression. Whereas some people with depression directly seek help from mental health professionals like psychologists and psychiatrists, this is not typical of most patients with depression. Many of them take the wait-and-see attitude and hope symptoms will go away on their own. Frequently, people with depression try some form of self-management, which may include cutting back on workload to allow more time to rest, change in lifestyles and diet, and trying out herbal medications. When these measures do not work, the next step is usually to seek help from their primary care physicians, the gate-keepers in the current health delivery system. In many countries, including the United States, primary care clinics are the de facto mental health services delivery system, particularly for the treatment of mood and anxiety disorders (Regier et al., 1978; Dolnak, 2006). Most depressed patients navigate by themselves in their help-seeking process. The health care delivery system and health professionals often tend to be passive participants in the recognition and the treatment of depression, which may explain in part the fact that depression is frequently under-recognized and under-treated in primary care (Williams et al., 1995; Katon et al., 1996). In fact, studies have shown that primary care physicians fail to recognize 30% to 50% of patients with depression (Simon & Von Korff, 1995).

The problems of untreated depression can be serious. People with untreated depression may experience loss of pleasurable feelings, a decline in quality of life, decreased productivity, impaired interpersonal relationships, and overeating and obesity, and may neglect their existing medical conditions due to a lack of motivation. This further results in people not adhering to the prescribed treatment for their conditions (Swenson et al., 2008; DeVellis & DeVellis, 2007). From a medical resource perspective, this generally means more clinical visits and higher medical costs (Katzelnick et al., 2000). In the worst-case scenario, patients with severe untreated depression could choose to end their suffering by committing suicide, a tragedy that frequently destroys family and social fabric (Fredman et al., 1988; Simon et al., 1995). Collaborative management of depression, with the involvement of a multidisciplinary team in primary care, may be an effective solution for improving the treatment of depression.

Many primary care physicians believe their main responsibility is to manage physical illnesses, which reflects the education they received during their medical training. Many of them do not feel equipped to handle mental illnesses (Gask et al., 2004), which are generally considered outside of their scope of services. Furthermore, the interviewing and handling of emotional problems frequently require longer visits, which go against the current climate of having shorter visits under managed care for the sake of efficiency and cost reduction. It has become inefficient, if not impossible, for primary care physicians to provide all necessary care in the limited time during outpatient visits. Hence there needs to be a collaborative approach to support the primary care physicians and to ensure that the patients who need treatment for depression are identified and offered appropriate treatment.

Collaborative management of depression in primary care

As described above, the need for a multidisciplinary treatment model is clear, as primary care clinics are often the gateways to treatment of depression, and primary care physicians often do not feel well equipped or are limited by managed care to treat mental illnesses effectively. Moreover, the seriousness of untreated depression cannot be denied. In Chapter 1, we introduced Wagner's (1998a) Chronic Care Model. This model emphasizes the need for a multidisciplinary approach to successfully manage chronic conditions in primary care settings. This model holds considerable promise for the treatment of patients with depression in primary care settings. The Chronic Care Model (Wagner, 1998a) involves multiple disciplines and a proactive approach to provide better services. The Chronic Care Model includes the establishment of a patient registry to provide active follow-up, population-based care, the adoption of treatment guidelines which have proven effectiveness for specific conditions, patient-centered collaborative goal-setting and self-management, planned and regular follow-up visits, and care management. In this comprehensive model, the two key activities are collaborative care and self-management education. The care manager, a relatively new member of the primary care team, plays a crucial role in both activities. Some clinics employ a nurse within the primary care team, while others use centralized care management services provided by an external agency to perform care management for their patients. The care manager "manages" patients according to an established protocol to provide health education, self-management skills, and greater intensity of care. They also facilitate communication with both the primary care doctors and supporting medical specialists and serve as the coordinator of the multidisciplinary team (Wagner, 1998a).

Based on the Chronic Care Model, Katon (1995) designed a collaborative model of treatment of depression in primary care, with the involvement of psychiatrists to provide consultation inside primary care clinics to depressed patients referred by primary care physicians. Psychiatrists and the primary care physicians jointly care for patients who require more intensive treatment than provided that by the primary care physicians alone. Katon's model also included intensive patient education and continued surveillance of adherence to medication regimens during the continuation and maintenance phases of treatment. He concluded that collaborative management resulted in more favorable outcomes in depression and improved satisfaction among patients with major depressive disorder (MDD).

The roles of care managers in the treatment of depression in primary care

As outlined in the Chronic Care Model and applied to the treatment of depression, care managers can perform a range of roles to improve the treatment of depression in primary care. These roles include systematic depression screening, individualized assessment of depressed patients, psychoeducation, setting treatment goals in collaboration with patients, training of problem-solving skills, coordination of care, and monitoring treatment outcomes.

Current status of active depression screening in primary care

An important hurdle in the early recognition of depression is that many people with depression are not aware of the condition. When patients do not actively seek help for their depression and when depression is not being recognized by their primary care physicians, treatment of depression is either non-existent or delayed. To improve recognition of depression, the US Preventive Services Task Force (USPSTF, 2002) recommends routine screening for depression in primary care settings that have systems in place to assure accurate diagnosis, effective treatment, and follow-up. In order to detect depression early, researchers in the past decades have studied depression screening instruments and found that many brief self-report questionnaires can readily identify depression. These questionnaires are usually symptom checklists which include the key symptoms of depression. In Table 2.1, we present information on four commonly used instruments for screening of depression: Beck Depression Inventory-II (BDI; Beck, Steer, & Brown, 1996); the 20-item Center for Epidemiological Studies Depression Scale (CES-D; Radloff, 1977); the 9-item Patient Health Questionnaire (PHQ-9; Kroenke & Spitzer, 2002); and the Quick Inventory of Depressive Symptomatology–Self-Report (QIDS-SR; Rush et al., 2006). All these questionnaires have been shown to be sensitive for detecting depression (high sensitivity) and accurate in not misdiagnosing people who do not have depression (high specificity). In general, these scales are designed to be accessible to patients with a sixth grade or higher education and can be completed within minutes. The development and the validation of a screening instrument is in fact an important step in the treatment of depression, as such instruments put an abstract concept of depression into a simple paper-pencil test for self-evaluation. Many of the depression screening instruments are now available online – several at no cost to the user – making it very convenient for people who have access to the Internet.

The screening instruments have provided the tools for early recognition of depression. However, the problem of under-recognition of depression has not been solved simply by having these instruments available. Most primary care clinics have yet to incorporate depression screening despite the availability of these instruments. There are many factors, including the lack of resources and technical difficulties in the implementation of depression screening, which will be described later in this chapter. Given that depression is a common condition in the primary clinic that is being under-recognized, care managers can facilitate early identification of depression by coordinating systematic depression screening in primary care clinics, perhaps through the use of these instruments.

The logistics of conducting depression screening are in fact more complex than it seems. One approach is for primary care physicians to have their patients fill out a screening questionnaire during clinical visits. Yet, the question follows regarding how often primary care physicians should administer screenings. To have primary care physicians screen for depression on all patients is expected to have a low yield, particularly if it is done on every visit, as the majority of patients do not have depression. To increase the efficiency of depression screening, some propose to screen those patients who report depressive symptoms or show observable signs of depression. Such an approach has been found to leave many patients with depression unrecognized, since people tend to under-report their depression, and many patients with depression express little signs of depression during a brief clinical visit. A more important challenge is that most primary

Table 2.1 Summary for clinicians of depression screening questionnaires

Measure	Number of items	Interpretation of scores	How to obtain a copy	Is there a fee for using this measure?
Center for Epidemiological Studies Depression Scale (CES-D)	20	15–21 = mild to moderate depression >21 = a high possibility of having MDD	http://med.stanford.edu/patienteducation/research/cesd.pdf	No
Patient Health Questionnaire (PHQ-9)	9	10–14 = mild depression 15–19 = moderate >19 = severe depression.	http://www.depression-primarycare.org/clinicians/toolkits/materials/forms/phq9/	No
Beck Depression Inventory (BDI) – II	21	0–13 = minimal depression 14–19 = mild depression 20–28 = moderate depression 29–63 = severe depression	http://pearsonassess.com/cgi-bin/MsmGo.exe?grab_id=0&page_id=593&query=beck&hiword=BECKER%20beck	Yes
Quick Inventory of Depressive Symptomatology-Self-Report (QIDS-SR)	16	6–10 = mild depression 11–15 = moderate depression 16–20 = severe >21 = very severe	http://www.ids-qids.org/	No

care physicians tend not to look for depression actively or consider treating depression beyond their scope of services.

The importance of depression screening in primary care clinics has received increasing attention in recent years. Since December 2007, the insurers of people with low income in Massachusetts (Medicaid) have mandated routine screening for behavioral problems, including depression, during annual check-ups for children and adolescents. It appears that it is a matter of time before such a requirement will extend to include adults as well as children, and will be followed by other insurers.

The role of care managers in facilitating depression screening

To reduce the workload on primary care physicians, care managers can play an important role in depression screening. They may coordinate with the clinic's support and nursing staff to distribute depression screening questionnaires, collect the completed questionnaires, and inform primary care physicians when patients screen positive for depression (i.e. report scores above an established cut-off score for that screening instrument). In some cases, people who screen positive for depression may not in fact have major depressive disorder, as many medical conditions have symptoms similar to those of depression. Subsequently, primary care physicians need to assess patients with positive screening results to determine whether they in fact have major depressive disorder and whether intervention is warranted. For patients who do not have major depressive disorder, their depressive symptoms usually remit after successful treatment of the medical conditions.

In many busy primary care clinics which serve a high volume of patients every day, systematic depression screening requires detailed record keeping and tracking of depression screening results. These administrative tasks could become a significant workload for the clinic staff, thus making depression screening an impractical and/or burdensome procedure. To circumvent this problem, some studies on depression screening in primary care had resorted to bundling depression screening with annual physical examination. Such an approach has been found to be effective and has been adopted in the primary care clinics under the Veterans Affairs (VA) hospital system. Some primary care clinics have their own mental health department or access to an affiliated mental health team. Care managers working in these clinics may seek support from the mental health team to provide the expertise and/or resources for depression screening and mental health consultations when appropriate.

The role of care managers in individualized assessment of depressed patients

Identifying patients with MDD is only the first step in the management of depression. To be able to engage a patient, it is important to find out how much the patient knows about depression and its treatment, whether or not he/she is willing to accept professional treatment, and the preferred choice of treatment if the patient is agreeable to receiving treatment. If the patient is ambivalent or reluctant to receive treatment for depression, the care manager should explore the reasoning behind such reluctance and address any misconceptions that may exist.

Many patients are skeptical of the diagnosis when they are informed of having MDD for the first time. Many consider their symptoms as part of normal or natural reaction to life stress. Some of them choose to manage their depression using willpower, even if they have already tried this approach for some time without success. Other patients consider a diagnosis of depression a sign of personal failure and worry about possible side effects of medications and the stigma associated with being labeled with a psychiatric condition. Lay people may have a totally different interpretation of depression than the medical and mental health professionals and pursue treatment approaches that are very different from those offered in conventional medicine settings. It is therefore important to understand patients' belief systems and treat them with respect so that the practitioner and the patient have a shared framework to communicate with each other. In any of these cases, educating patients about depression and its treatment is the first step to engage patients and to inform them about available treatment options.

The role of care managers in depression education

Many practitioners assume that patients know a lot about depression and that it would be redundant to offer a full description and explanation. While this may be true for many patients, it is not true for others, particularly for people coming from non-Western cultural backgrounds that traditionally put less emphasis on psychological problems. Care managers can play a crucial role in educating patients about depression, as most primary care practitioners are unable to do it during clinical visits.

While the cause of depression is not completely understood, the prevalent viewpoint held by the scientific community is that multiple factors are involved, including genetics, early childhood adversity, and stressful life events, as well as the relative absence of social support networks. While the relative weights or influence of each of these factors may vary from person to person, clinicians have also observed that patients frequently make their own attributions on what may have caused their depression. Part of the care managers' training is to be able to align themselves with patients' understanding so that they can successfully engage them in treatment. Many patients find the monoamine theory of depression, which hypothesizes that depression is due to a relative deficiency of monoamines and their activity in the brain, a useful framework for understanding the biological basis of depression, even though this theory is considered by researchers to be obsolete and probably overly simplistic. Such a framework, however, does provide a simple rationale for taking antidepressant medications as an antidote for their depression. Care managers should educate the patients that current treatment guidelines (APA, 2000a) state that the best treatment for depression varies according to its severity; for mild and moderate depression, specific psychotherapeutic interventions including cognitive behavioral therapy (CBT) and interpersonal therapy (IPT) are as effective as antidepressant medications. For severe depression, medication treatment with or without psychotherapy is typically considered the treatment of choice. Yet more recent studies suggest that CBT is equally as effective as antidepressant medications in patients with more severe depression (Feldman, 2007). With this understanding, patients are encouraged to decide on their preferred method of treatment.

The care manager should inform patients that the average untreated episode of depression typically lasts 5 months (APA, 2000b) but can stretch on for years. This explains why medications should not be stopped when depression symptoms begin to subside, as the risk for relapse may persist well beyond the acute phase. Patients should also be informed that, when they are started on antidepressant treatment, it may take up to 4 to 6 weeks before they experience significant clinical improvement. With such an understanding, patients do not become disappointed and drop out of treatment when they observe only little improvement in the first few weeks of treatment. If patients experience a lack of response to medication after a trial of sufficient duration, care managers can inform patients that other options may be available, including switching to a second medication or adding psychotherapy or other medications. Even if they do not see improvements, patients should also be discouraged from discontinuing medication without consulting with their physician, as abrupt termination of some medication can produce very unpleasant symptoms.

While primary care physicians are responsible for educating patients about medications, care managers can be an invaluable resource to review the information and to offer patients the opportunity for further discussion. The care manager should clarify the benefits of medication treatment as well as the common side effects of antidepressant medications. Patients should anticipate possible side effects, including dyspepsia, nausea, constipation, diarrhea, sleepiness, fatigue, anxiety, and sexual dysfunction, and be reassured that many of these side effects tend to become less intense after several weeks. Because different antidepressant medications have different side effect profiles, care managers should guide patients in selecting their medications of choice, based on their tolerability profile, under the supervision of the physician in the team. Care managers should also inform patients that, in rare occasions, antidepressants could lead to suicidal thoughts and impulses among children, adolescents, and young adults; thus patients should notify the treatment team immediately when this happens.

Some patients worry that they could become physically or psychologically dependent on antidepressants once they are started on the medications. Care managers should reassure patients that antidepressants in general do not cause dependency. Long-term medication treatment is sometimes needed for patients with recurrent depression. This is intended to reduce the chance of relapse of depression, and this should not be misinterpreted as a form of physical or psychological dependency. Therefore, a return of depressive symptoms may occur in the context of premature discontinuation of treatment.

Some patients are reluctant to accept treatment in fear of being stigmatized for having a "mental condition." Care managers may guide them to weigh the pros and cons of having versus not having treatment; the latter carries the risk of significant personal distress, as well as impairment in interpersonal, social, and occupational functioning. Psychoeducation provides the relevant information for patients with depression to help them make informed decisions and to discard the fears and misconceptions about the disease and its treatment, and introduces the skills for self-management of mood symptoms.

To facilitate education about depression, several institutions have developed depression toolkits that contain pertinent information about depression. Some of the information is intended for patients, and other toolkits are for primary care physicians. The depression toolkit developed by the McArthur Foundation (http://www.depression-primarycare.org/clinicians/toolkits/full/) is available online, providing useful information about depression. Helpful informational resources are also available in English and Spanish from the National Institute of Mental Health (http://www.nimh.nih.gov/health/topics/depression/index.shtml). An interactive tutorial with self-scoring comprehension questions is also available in English and Spanish (http://www.nlm.nih.gov/medlineplus/depression.html). Another useful website was developed by the British Columbia Partners for Mental Health and Addictions Information (http://www.heretohelp.bc.ca/skills/managing-depression). These depression toolkits can be used by care managers as readily available teaching materials for depression. It is hoped that these useful informational resources will be translated into different languages to benefit more patients from diverse cultural backgrounds.

Other key aspects of care management beyond screening, assessment, and education

In the earlier parts of the chapter, we explained the importance of active screening for early identification of depression, preparing patients for individualized treatment, and educating patients and families about the nature of depression. We also propose that beyond these roles, case managers can be instrumental in helping patients fully benefit from treatment throughout the various stages of treatment, including initial assessment and diagnosis, to symptom reduction, and eventual relapse prevention. What case managers provide to patients is ultimately multifaceted. Case managers utilize different techniques grounded in psychological theories and approaches to best understand and provide what each patient needs in order to seek, accept, and utilize treatment for depression. Care managers also help provide the necessary follow-up and support to maintain treatment gains. In the spirit of multidisciplinary care, care managers draw from a variety of approaches and techniques toward the ultimate goal of treating depression and enhancing the overall psychological and physical well-being of patients.

Collaborative goal-setting: the use of motivational interviewing

In a previous study on systematic depression screening in a primary care clinic which focuses on serving Asian immigrants (Yeung et al., 2006), our team encountered a hurdle that was unanticipated. When patients who screened positive for depression were informed of the results of their screening, a substantial proportion of them remained unconvinced or uncertain about having depression. Some tried to explain the screening outcome as usual sadness associated with problems in their lives or minimized the symptoms as part of their personality. They were ambivalent or unready about making changes in their lifestyles, resetting their priorities in life, or accepting the recommendation of psychotherapy or antidepressant treatment. Part of the care manager's role is to point out to these patients the need to take action, and that patients are capable of making positive change in their lives. To motivate patients, care managers can help the patient envision how things might be if change did happen and help them see the light at the end of the tunnel. Motivational interviewing is an interview technique that can be very useful to persuade patients to accept treatments that are proven useful for their conditions.

As we discussed in Chapter 1, motivational interviewing was initially designed for approaching patients with substance abuse problems who are not yet ready for change. It was later adopted for use in changing the behaviors of people with chronic diseases. It is a directive, patient-centered counseling style for eliciting behavior change by helping patients explore and resolve ambivalence.

The focus of motivational interviewing is on eliciting the person's intrinsic motivation for change. It does not impose changes as an authority. Rather, it elicits motivation from within the patient (Miller & Rollnick, 2002). This is usually achieved by discussing with the person the disadvantages of the status quo (e.g. having significant depression symptoms) and the advantages of change (e.g. the remission of depression symptoms and improvement in functioning).

The four general principles of motivational interviewing (MI) are as follows:
(1) Express empathy
(2) Develop a discrepancy
(3) Tolerate resistance
(4) Support self-efficacy

To express empathy in MI means to be able to understand and accept the patient's experience, including the patient's ambivalence towards change. To develop a discrepancy is to use skills to help patients become aware of the inconsistencies between the patient's present behavior and important personal goals or values to motivate the patient to change. It is more effective for the provider to help patients identify the discrepancies, and not to identify the discrepancy for the patient. The principle of tolerating resistance is important so that care managers do not impose their own views and confront the resistance from the patient. Instead, they should bring up questions and invite patients to come up with their own answers and solutions. To support self-efficacy, care managers communicate to patients the belief in the possibility of change, emphasize the patients' ability to change, and encourage the patients to choose and carry out a plan to change their behavior (Levensky et al., 2007).

There are four basic skills that are frequently used in MI:

(1) Reflective listening
(2) Asking open questions
(3) Affirming
(4) Summarizing

Reflective listening is the skill of stating back to the patient a specific part or aspect of his/her statement. In doing so, the provider tries to acknowledge the patient's thoughts and feelings, clarify whether he/she understands the statement correctly, and selectively reiterate the statements the patient makes that are in favor of change. Reflection can be simply repeating or elaborating part of what the patient has said. Although it sounds simplistic, reflection is effective in building rapport and facilitating movement in the direction of change.

Care managers ask open questions to bring up discussion of the reasons for making desired changes. By asking questions, the care manager encourages the patient to explore the discrepancies between what his/her goals are and the current behavior. The exercise of processing ideas, verbalizing them, and putting them in writing helps many patients "face" their thoughts and solidify their awareness and motivation for change. Asking open questions instead of offering direct advice and direction is extremely helpful in reducing resistance from patients regarding change.

Affirming is based on the principle of behavioral therapy that specific behaviors increase if they are being reinforced or rewarded. Affirming can be done by directly showing support for the patient's efforts and success in accomplishing his/her goals. It is an important skill in promoting patient confidence and is effective in enhancing patient self-efficacy. Sometimes expressing affirmation by acknowledging efforts made by the patient can mobilize him or her to continue taking steps to address depressive symptoms.

The care manager may offer a summary statement by summing up the important elements of what the patient has said to help the patient see what has been accomplished and the challenges ahead, and then to discuss the next steps in reaching the set goals.

Motivational interviewing is based on the spirit of collaboration. The care manager may use MI to persuade patients to follow his/her recommendation, instead of using an authoritative stance to coerce change. The goal is to elicit or draw out the motivation for change from within the person and to respect the person's autonomy. It emphasizes that the responsibility and the decision for change are left with the person, and the change serves the person's own goals and values. Motivational interviewing has been shown to be more effective than traditional advice giving in modifying behavior related to the prevention and treatment of a broad range of diseases, and this technique is also effective in health education initiatives such as substance abuse counseling, HIV risk reduction, adherence to diet and exercise, and health-safety practices (Miller & Rollnick, 2002).

Skills enhancement: the use of problem-solving therapy

Problem-solving therapy was originally developed for the treatment of depression. However, it has since been applied to helping people adjust to a variety of stressful experiences, including medical conditions. As such, an appeal of this approach is that it can help normalize treatment for depression in that it can be presented to clients as a means of optimizing personal skills for setting goals and dealing effectively with problems, which are a universal experience. It can be thought of as a conscious, rational effort by which a person attempts to identify or discover effective or adaptive solutions for specific problems encountered in daily living (D'Zurilla and Nuzu, 2007).

In the social problem-solving model proposed by D'Zurilla and Nezu (1999), the outcomes of problem solving are determined by two independent processes: problem orientation and problem-solving skills. Problem orientation involves the recognition that there is a problem, which could be physical symptoms, psychological distress, marital and family problems, work-related problems, or any problems that exist in the person's life. Having recognized the existence of a problem, the person then assesses the problem and finds out the cause of the problem.

Problem orientation

Problem orientation is the ability of a person to be aware of and to understand the problems at hand and his or her own problem-solving ability. It is a thinking process that involves the following:
(a) the appraisal of a problem as a challenge,
(b) the belief that problems are solvable,
(c) belief in one's ability to solve problems successfully (problem-solving efficacy),

(d) belief that successful problem solving takes time and effort, and
(e) committing oneself to solving problems rather than avoiding them (D'Zurilla and Nuzu, 2007).

Problem orientation is a very important process in problem solving because it is the point at which a person assesses the importance of the problem and decides on the extent of mobilization and resource allocation to solve a given problem. The care managers, with their professional training and understanding of depression, can play a very important role when patients form their problem orientation. They can guide patients to pay attention to problems that affect their mood in a positive and negative way and to recognize their depressive symptoms and how they have an impact on their lives so that sufficient time and energy will be allocated to addressing the symptoms. Care managers may model positive problem orientation towards a problem. They can help patients to view their problem as an opportunity for personal growth or self-improvement and to understand that they are able to solve the problem on their own. With such an orientation, patients can focus on constructive problem-solving activities, maximize effort and persistence, and be more able to tolerate frustration and uncertainty in the course of overcoming their problems. Care managers may also encourage patients to be flexible; when they have tried their best and still cannot succeed, they may consider viewing the problem from a different perspective, either to accept it, seek a compromise, or get help to overcome it.

Problem-solving skills

Once the problem is identified, a care manager will assist patients with problem-solving skills to define the most pertinent problem and to avoid using irrational or magical thinking, which tends to distort the nature of the problem. According to the model proposed by D'Zurilla and Nuzu (2007), there are four major problem-solving skills: They are:

(1) Problem definition and formulation
(2) Generation of alternative solutions
(3) Decision making
(4) Solution implementation and verification

The skill of problem definition and formulation is the ability to gather relevant and factual information about the problem, identify the nature of the problem, and set a realistic problem-solving goal. For patients with depression, this refers to the recognition of symptoms of depression, the understanding of the nature of depression and available treatment, and the formation of a problem-solving goal. There are two important rules in goal-setting: the goal needs to be stated in specific, concrete terms and should be realistic and attainable. Setting a specific, concrete goal helps to shape the appropriate solutions and how to measure whether the approaches are effective. For example, the goal to reduce the number of overdue assignments in a week is a more objective and measurable goal than to "become a better employee." Similarly, to increase the number of hours to be spent with one's spouse is a more concrete goal than "to improve marital relationship." The importance of setting realistic goals is apparent, as unachieved goals lead to disappointment and frustration.

Cost-effectiveness analysis is a useful approach to formulating solutions, and many people do it intuitively for problem solving. It can be done in a systematic way by listing the benefits and costs of solving the problem and the costs and benefits if a set goal is being achieved. For instance, a clinician could ask a client to imagine what life would be like if this problem were resolved and what life would be like if a person decided to take no action to change the situation. A simple exercise like this can be extremely helpful in the appraisal process and may shed light on seemingly complex and difficult problems.

The skill to generate alternative solutions is to produce a list of potential solutions to maximize the chances of including the best solution. It is a good habit to avoid using knee-jerk reactions in coming up with solutions. Frequently, the first idea that comes to mind may not be the most feasible and effective approach for problem solving. It is generally beneficial to take time to "brainstorm" possible solutions, even ones that may not be perfect or even realistic, as they may lead to other effective solutions. Care managers may help patients explore alternative solutions or suggest relevant resources like books and experts to help them generate as many different solutions as possible and pick the best one from a variety of potential solutions.

To facilitate the process of decision making, care managers may help patients decide and choose among available solutions based on their experience and their understanding about depression. They may offer their predictions on possible outcomes and consequences of the possible solutions and point out which option has the potential to give the best outcomes and which of the alternatives are less feasible or more likely to have serious negative consequences. To appraise the relative merits of the alternatives, D'Zurilla and Nezu (2007) suggest evaluating each of the alternatives using these four questions:

(1) Will this solution solve the problem?
(2) Can I really carry it out?
(3) What are the overall effects on myself, both short-term and long-term?
(4) What are the overall effects on others, both short-term and long-term?

The answers to these four questions generally help decision making from the available alternatives.

After the patient has made his/her decision and implemented the solution, the care manager will assess with the patient the outcomes and whether the problems have been adequately resolved. If the goal that was set was a concrete and measurable goal, this is a relatively straightforward and easy step, simply by checking if the goal has been attained.

Follow-up and support

After the patient has been engaged and started on medication and/or psychotherapy, care managers maintain an important role to follow up and provide support. They actively contact patients periodically to encourage them to stay on treatment for depression since many patients may decide to prematurely stop their treatment in the initial months (Sonawalla et al., 2002). Ideally, care managers remain available to patients through telephone contacts for questions on depression and medication treatment and side effects. In addition to providing information, they can also provide reassurance and problem-solving treatment to problems that arise and monitor treatment outcomes using instruments such as those presented in Table 2.1. If a patient fails to show up at a scheduled visit to the primary care physician, the care manager can contact the patient to inquire why he/she missed the appointment. When a patient does not respond well to treatment, the care manager may seek input from the consultant psychiatrist and may communicate the recommendation to the patient's primary care physician. If necessary, the care manager can arrange a psychiatric consultation for patients with more complicated depressions (e.g. major psychiatric comorbidity or past treatment failures) or if the depression is refractory to treatment. Follow-up and support is important for generalization of treatment gains, solidifying skill sets learned from treatment, and overall relapse prevention.

The IMPACT Study: an example of collaborative management of depression in primary care

In the following paragraphs, we will describe the Improving Mood-Promoting Access to Collaborative Treatment (IMPACT) Study (Unützer et al., 2002), one of the key studies to evaluate the effectiveness of collaborative management in primary care clinics. In this study, older patients with late-life depression were recruited from primary care clinics and randomly assigned to receive either active intervention (collaborative care for depression) or usual care. Those who received collaborative care for depression were sent a 20-minute educational videotape and a booklet about late-life depression and were encouraged to have an initial visit with a care manager at the primary care clinic. It was postulated that collaborative management of depression with the use of intensive patient contact and monitoring, specialized staff training, standardized treatment algorithm, and the network of supervisory support would provide the needed resources to improve the outcomes of patients who were treated for depression in the primary care setting.

In this study, care managers were nurses or psychologists who had received training to become depression clinical specialists. During their initial 60-minute visit with the patients, the care managers reviewed the patients' medical history, family structure, and their relevant interpersonal relationships. They also encouraged patients to become active participants in their depression care.

Care managers also discussed with patients educational materials sent to them and asked their preferences for depression treatment, which were generally a choice between taking an antidepressant medication or a course of six- to eight-session problem-solving therapy delivered by the care manager. The treatment plan was finalized and decided by the patient and his/her regular primary care practitioner. Care managers also encouraged patients to schedule pleasant life events and referred them to additional health or social services as clinically indicated. During the course of depression treatment, care managers obtained supervision from a psychiatrist and a liaison primary care practitioner in the team and stayed in contact with patients for up to 12 months to monitor their treatment response with a standard instrument. Care managers also tracked whether patients attended their primary care physicians' regular follow-up visits. During the first 6 months of treatment, care managers either met with patients in person or contacted them using telephone calls on a weekly or biweekly basis. After patients had improved and their symptoms had subsided, care managers would engage the patient to develop a relapse prevention plan and to maintain contact with them on a monthly basis. If a patient's symptoms worsened or became unresponsive to medication or problem-solving treatment, the care manager would consult with the supervising team psychiatrist, who was available to see the patients if necessary. For patients with more severe depression, the psychiatrist could recommend a higher level of treatment if necessary. Based on the findings collected from a wide range of participating primary care clinics, the researchers of the IMPACT Study concluded that the Collaborative Care Model was feasible and more effective than usual care for depression.

Additional empirical support for collaborative management of depression in primary care

In 2006, Hunkeler et al. performed a follow-up study on the subjects of the IMPACT study and showed that 1 year after IMPACT resources were withdrawn, depressed patients who had received collaborative care continued to show better depression outcomes, suggesting that collaborative care for depressed elderly adults had lasting beneficial effects. Gilbody and colleagues (2003) published a narrative systematic review on educational and organizational interventions to improve the management of depression in primary care. They concluded that effective interventions were those with complex interventions that incorporated clinician education, care management, and integration between primary and secondary care. They also pointed out that simple guideline implementation and education strategies were likely to be ineffective. They concluded that to provide effective intervention for depression in primary care, substantial investment is needed in primary care services and a major shift in the organization and provision of care. Later, Gilbody et al. (2006a) performed a cumulative meta-analysis on the long-term outcomes from 37 randomized studies on collaborative management of depression in primary care and concluded that collaborative care is a more effective model than usual care for both shorter (6 months) and longer (up to 5 years) terms.

Trying to address the question of how to improve depression treatment on a large scale, Simon et al. (2004) investigated a telephone intervention to provide both care management and cognitive behavioral psychotherapy to depressed primary care patients beginning antidepressant treatment. The researchers showed that such a program improves satisfaction and clinical outcomes. They concluded that this could be a new public health model for active outreach to provide psychotherapy for depression.

There are several interesting cost-benefit analysis studies on collaborative treatment of depression in primary care. Gilbody et al. (2006b) conducted a systematic review of randomized economic evaluations and concluded that improved outcomes from collaborative care required the investment of additional cost. They estimated that the cost for a depression-free day ranged from £7 to £13. In the same study, they found that use of educational interventions alone were associated with increased cost and no clinical benefit. In the same year, Wang et al. (2006) published a cost-effectiveness and cost-benefit analysis on screening and depression care management for workers and found that it required an incremental cost of $19,976 for each quality-adjusted life-year relative to usual care, and that such a cost is within the range for medical interventions usually covered by employer-sponsored insurance. This study concluded that enhanced depression care yields a net cumulative benefit of $2,895 after 5 years as a result of increased worker productivity. In 2007, Wang et al. studied a program for telephone screening, outreach, and care management for depressed workers. They found that a systematic program to identify depression and promote effective treatment improves not only clinical outcomes, but also workplace outcomes. Depressed workers who received the intervention from the program had higher job retention and worked more hours than the usual care group. The researchers concluded that many employers would in fact experience a positive return on investing in such treatment programs, since the investment expense can be recovered from hiring, training, and salary costs.

Barriers in implementing collaborative care for depression in primary care

Despite the fact that adequate evidence from research shows that depression screening and care management improve outcomes in the treatment of depression and is cost effective over a 5-year period, collaborative management of depression has only been infrequently implemented in most primary care settings. It has been shown repeatedly that after the completion of collaborative management research projects, most primary care clinics reverted to the old system of usual care. This indicates that there are significant barriers under the current health delivery system in implementing collaborative management of depression in primary care. These barriers of implementation can be categorized as technical difficulties, the practice orientation of primary care physicians, and reimbursement policy of insurers.

Technical difficulties

There are lingering technical or logistical issues in implementing the collaborative model which have not been completely resolved. Different primary care clinics have different staffing structures and, currently, most primary care clinics do not have care managers. The question arises regarding who should perform depression screening – whether it should be the physician, the nursing staff, support staff, or the patients themselves. Nowadays, depression screening tools are easily accessible online, and more and more patients are familiar with the usefulness of depression screening. It is hoped that patients can play a more active role in depression screening to lower the cost and labor involved in the process. Even so, the primary care clinic will still need to provide the administrative support so that it is done in a systematic manner. In many studies, depression specialists were trained to function as care managers. In actual clinical practice, it would be unrealistic to have a single specialist for each of the common medical and mental disorders, including diabetes, hypertension, arthritis, anxiety, depression, and substance abuse. Most clinical staff do not have the expertise to provide specialized care managers for all of these disorders. To resolve this problem, new education programs need to be established to train people who are able to perform care management for a wide variety of disorders. There are also remaining questions on whether all patients with depression need care management or whether only certain patients would benefit from care management, and how to tailor the content and duration of psychoeducation, MI, problem-solving therapy, and follow-up supports to fit the needs of each individual patient.

The practice orientation of primary care physicians

The second barrier is the practice habits of the primary care physicians – whether they consider identification and treatment of depression an integral part of their clinical work or the treatment of depression as the responsibility of mental health professionals. In the current health delivery system, it is inevitable that primary care physicians and mental health providers work hand-in-hand in recognizing and in treating depression. In the past decade, primary care physicians have been increasingly aware of the problem of untreated depression in their practice and have been more involved in the treatment of depression. Nevertheless, there is much to be done to put in place a systematic effort in depression screening, in providing education, support, monitoring, and self-management training to patients with depression.

Reimbursement policy of insurers

The third barrier is the lack of resources in implementing depression screening and collaborative management. Both depression screening and care management involve the investment of additional costs, and there are no resources for these activities unless they are supported by research funding. Most insurers reimburse services provided in primary care clinics based on the number of clinic encounters or visits, and depression screening and care management typically obtain no reimbursement. Subsequently, there are little incentives for primary care clinics to continue such activities after the research is completed. Recently, some insurers have started to pay attention to the importance of quality of care and have started to provide incentives for activities that lead to improved clinical outcomes. Yet the incentives continue to be symbolic and not enough to modify the current form of "usual care."

Conclusion

With the development of newer antidepressants with less side effects and effective psychotherapeutic interventions, most patients with depression can benefit from medical treatment if they are readily identified and treated. Systematic depression screening in the primary care and care management have been shown to be an effective model for improving treatment of depression, and the collaborative management model provides long-term clinical benefits. The importance of such a collaborative model has received increasing support from research. Educating the public about the importance of recognition and adequate treatment of depression, training primary care physicians to take on increased responsibilities in the treatment of depression, educating medical staff to have care management expertise, and influencing public opinion and legislation to pressure insurers to pay for depression screening and care management are all effective means to improve treatment of depression. Some insurers have started to offer care management for severe mental disorders and are extending these services to include patients with depression. There are signs that screening for behavioral problems may emerge as routine practice. As noted previously, in November 2007, Medicaid, the insurer for patients with low income in Massachusetts, has mandated all pediatricians to screen for behavioral problems, including depression, during annual examinations for children and adolescents.

It is anticipated that systematic screening and care management for depressed patients may gain more acceptance and momentum in the coming years.

REFERENCES

American Psychiatric Association. Practice guidelines for the treatment of patients with major depressive disorder (revision). *Am J Psychiatry*. 2000a; 157:1–45.

American Psychiatric Association. Diagnostic and Statistical Manual of Mental Disorders. 4th edn, text revision. Washington, DC: American Psychiatric Association; 2000b.

Baer L, Jacobs DG, Meszler-Reizes J, Blais M, Fava M, Kessler R, Magruder K, Murphy J, Kopans B, Cukor P, Leahy L, O'Laughlen J. Development of a brief screening instrument: the HANDS. *Psychother Psychosom*. 2000; 69:35–41.

Beck AT, Steer RA, Brown GK. Manual for the Beck Depression Inventory-II. San Antonio, TX: Psychological Corporation; 1996.

DeVellis BM, DeVellis RF. Depression and arthritis. *N C Med J*. 2007; 68(6):434–435.

Dolnak DR. Treating patients for comorbid depression, anxiety disorders, and somatic illnesses. *J Am Osteopath Assoc*. 2006 106(5 Suppl 2):S1–8.

Dowrick C, Dixon C, Sutton C, Perry R, Torgerson D, Usherwood T. A pragmatic cluster randomized controlled trial of an educational intervention for GPs in the assessment and management of depression. *Psychol Med*. 2004; 34(1):63–72.

D'Zurilla TJ, Nezu AM. Problem-Solving Therapy: A Social Competence Approach in Clinical Intervention. 2nd edn. New York, NY: Springer; 1999.

D'Zurilla TJ, Nezu AM. Problem-Solving Therapy: A Positive Approach to Clinical Intervention. 3rd edn. New York, NY: Springer; 2007.

Feldman GC. Cognitive and behavioral therapies for depression: overview, new directions, and practical recommendations for dissemination. *Psychiatr Clin North Am*. 2007; 30(1):39–50.

Fredman L, Weissman MM, Leaf PJ, Bruce ML. Social functioning in community residents with depression and other psychiatric disorders: results of the New Haven Epidemiologic Catchment Area study. *J Affect Disord*. 1988; 15:103–112.

Gask L, Dowrick C, Dixon C, Sutton C, Perry R, Torgerson D, Usherwood T. A pragmatic cluster randomized controlled trial of an educational intervention for GPs in the assessment and management of depression. *Psychol Med*. 2004; 34(1):63–72.

Gilbody S, Whitty P, Grimshaw J, Thomas R. Education and organizational interventions to improve the management of depression in primary care. *JAMA*. 2003; 289:3145–3151.

Gilbody S, Bower P, Fletcher J, Richards D, Sutton AJ. Collaborative Care for Depression: a cumulative meta-analysis and review of longer-term outcomes. *Arch Intern Med*. 2006a; 166:2314–2321.

Gilbody S, Bower P, Whitty P. Costs and consequences of enhanced primary care for depression: systematic review of randomized economic evaluations. *Brit J Psychiatry*. 2006b; 189:297–308.

Hunkeler EM, Katon W, Tang L, Williams JW Jr, Kroenke K, Lin EH, Harpole LH, Arean P, Levine S, Grypma LM, Hargreaves WA, Unützer J. Long term outcomes form the

IMPACT randomized trial for depressed elderly patients in primary care. BMJ. 2006; 332:259–263.

Katon W, Korff MV, Lin E, Walker E, Simon G, Bush T, Robinson P, Russo J. Collaborative management to achieve treatment guidelines: impact on depression in primary care. *JAMA*. 1995; 273:1026–1031.

Katon W, Robinson P, Von Korff Michael, Lin E, Bush T, Ludman E, Simon G, Walker E. A multifaceted intervention to improve treatment of depression in primary care. *Arch Gen Psychiatry*. 1996; 53:924–932.

Katzelnick DJ, Simon GE, Pearson SD, Manning WG, Helstad CP, Henk HJ, Cole SM, Lin EH, Taylor LH, Kobak KA. Randomized trial of a depression management program in high utilizers of medical care. *Arch Fam Med*. 2000; 9(8):689–670.

Kroenke K, Spitzer RL. The PHQ-9: a new depression diagnostic and severity measure. *Psychiatr Ann*. 2002; 9:1–7.

Levensky ER, Forcehimes A, O'Donohue WT, Beitz K. Motivational interviewing: an evidence-based approach to counseling helps patients follow treatment recommendations. *Am Nurs. 2007*; 107:50–58.

Miller WR, Rollnick S. Motivational Interviewing: Preparing People for Change. 2nd edn. New York, NY: Guilford Press; 2002.

Radloff LS (1977). The CES-D scale: a self report depression scale for research in the general population. *Appl Psychol Meas*. 1977; 1:385–401.

Regier DA, Goldberg ID, Taube CA. The de facto US mental health services system: a public health perspective. *Arch Gen Psychiatry*. 1978; 35(6):685–693.

Rush AJ, Carmody TJ, Ibrahim HM, Trivedi MH, Biggs MM, Shores-Wilson K, Crismon ML, Toprac MG, Kashner TM. Comparison of self-report and clinician ratings on two inventories of depressive symptomatology. *Psychiatr Serv*. 2006; 57(6):829–837.

Simon GE, Von Korff M. Recognition, management, and outcomes of depression in primary care. *Arch Fam Med*. 1995; 4:99–105.

Simon GE, Von Korff M, Barlow W. Health care costs of primary care patients with recognized depression. *Arch Gen Psychiatry*. 1995; 52:850–856.

Simon GE, Ludman EJ, Tutty S, Operskalski B, Von Korff M. Telephone psychotherapy and telephone care management for primary care patients starting antidepressant treatment: a randomized controlled trial. *JAMA*. 2004; 292:935–942.

Sonawalla SB, Farabaugh AH, Leslie VM, Pava JA, Matthews JD, Fava M. Early drop-outs, late drop-outs and completers: differences in the continuation phase of a clinical trial. *Prog Neuropsychopharmacol Biol Psychiatry*. 2002; 26(3):415–419.

Swenson SL, Rose M, Vittinghoff E, Stewart A, Schillinger D. The influence of depressive symptoms on clinician-patient communication among patients with type 2 diabetes. *Med Care*. 2008; 46(3):257–265

United States Preventive Services Task Force (USPSTF) . Depression Screening. 2002. Available at http://www.ahrq.gov/clinic/uspstf/uspsdepr.htm

Unützer J, Katon W, Callahan CM, Williams JW Jr, Hunkeler E, Harpole L, Hoffing M, Della Penna RD, Noël PH, Lin EH, Areán PA, Hegel MT, Tang L, Belin TR, Oishi S, Langston C; IMPACT Investigators. Collaborative care management of late-life depression in the primary care setting: a randomized controlled trial. *JAMA*. 2002; 288:2836–2845.

Wagner EH. More than a case manager. *Ann Intern Med*. 1998a; 129:654–656.

Wagner EH. Chronic disease management: what will it take to improve care for chronic illness? *Eff Clin Pract.* 1998b; 1:2–4.

Wang PS, Patrick, A, Avorn J, Azocar F, Ludman E, McCulloch J, Simon G, Kessler R. The costs and benefits of enhanced depression care to employers. *Arch Gen Psychiatry.* 2006; 63:1345–1353.

Wang PS, Simon GE, Avorn J, Azocar F, Ludman EJ, McCulloch J, Petukhova MZ, Kessler RC. Telephone screening, outreach, and care management for depressed workers and impact on clinical and work productivity outcomes: a randomized controlled trial. *JAMA.* 2007; 298:1401–1411.

Williams JW, Kerber CA, Mulrow C, Medina A, Aguilar C. Depressive disorders in primary care: prevalence, functional disability, and identification. *J Gen Intern Med.* 1995; 10:7–12.

Yeung AS, Yu SC, Fung F, Vorono S, Fava M. Recognizing and engaging depressed Chinese Americans in treatment in a primary care setting. *Int J Geriatr Psychiatry.* 2006; 21:819–823.

Self-assessment instruments for depression

Introduction

Modern medicine has reaped the benefit of technological advances to provide objective measures for the diagnosis of medical diseases and for monitoring treatment response. For example, patients who suffer from diabetes can measure their blood sugar as an index to gauge the severity of the disease and its response to treatment, and, similarly, patients with hypertension can measure their blood pressure at home. However, similar objective measurements are yet to be found for psychiatric disorders. Clinicians who treat patients with depression and other psychiatric disorders continue to rely on patients' self-reports of their symptoms, distress, and functional impairment to both identify the illness and to monitor its response to treatment.

The reliance on patients' self-reports has obvious drawbacks; during clinical visits, patients tend to report what they consider most urgent, and patients' reports are often influenced by the perception of their illnesses. Similarly, clinicians trained in different health disciplines may focus on specific aspects of the provided information, which are related to their own backgrounds, to help them conceptualize the illness and formulate an intervention using pharmacological, psychodynamic, cognitive, behavioral, or interpersonal approaches. In the absence of satisfactory laboratory tests to measure the severity of depression, standardized clinician-rated and self-assessment instruments are the most reliable and objective outcome measurement tools for depression. The use of standardized instruments in clinical and research interviews provides a more consistent approach to elicit psychological symptoms in a way that is less affected by the patients' and the clinicians' orientation. Clinical data collected with use of standardized instruments have increased reliability, a prerequisite for high-quality scientific research, compared with those collected through unstructured clinician-rated interviews. It is based on the changes in the depression scores of these instruments that the efficacy of specific interventions for depression, including biological, pharmacological, and psychological treatments, are determined. Thus far, researchers tend to give preference to clinician-rated instruments over self-assessment instruments due to the perceived limitations of the latter, including a reduced sensitivity to detect change. Yet self-assessment instruments have gained increasing acceptance. Two of the self-report instruments that we will discuss in a later section of this chapter (Inventory of Depressive Symptomatology–Self-Report [IDS-SR] and Quick Inventory of Depressive Symptomatology Self-Report [QIDS-SR]) were recently accepted by the US Food and Drug Administration (FDA) as valid outcome measurement instruments in clinical trials on depression, a decision based on the available data in support of the instruments' psychometric properties. In this chapter, we will focus on the use of standardized self-rated instruments for major depressive disorder (MDD). To be consistent with other chapters of the book, we will continue to use the lay term "depression" for MDD. This is also consistent with self-rated instruments that measure severity of depression symptoms rather than making a categorical diagnosis of MDD.

Compared with clinician-rated instruments, self-rated instruments have several advantages: they are less time-consuming and less expensive to administer, they do not require trained personnel for administration, and they do not suffer from potential biases introduced by the observations and subjective judgments of clinicians. Self-assessment instruments are also useful for eliciting the patient's perception of his/her own illness and degree of recovery. Self-assessment is highly consistent with the goals of self-management. It allows patients to monitor their symptom severity outside of contact with clinicians, allowing patients to track improvement and detect symptom worsening. This feedback can inform patients' use of self-management strategies discussed in later chapters.

In the first part of the chapter, we will discuss the properties of good self-assessment instruments for monitoring the severity of depression, the evolution of the concept of depression in the past five decades, and its impact on the development of self-rated instruments, followed by the introduction of several self-assessment instruments for depression that are widely used in clinical studies. In the second part of the chapter, we will discuss the validity indices of screening instruments, the applications of these self-rated instruments for depression screening, the effectiveness of depression screening, and the importance of depression screening in the primary care setting. In the final section, we address the role clinicians play in the use of self-assessment instruments both for screening and for self-monitoring of symptoms by presenting practical considerations of how to integrate such instruments in research and clinical practice.

Properties of self-assessment instruments for monitoring severity of depression

Many scales have been developed to measure symptoms of depression. A good instrument for depression should have certain psychometric properties, such as high reliability and validity. In terms of testing reliability of self-report depression questionnaires, researchers typically focus on internal consistency of its items (i.e. high correlation amongst the items). There are several types of validity for measuring instruments. Most broadly, construct validity refers to how well the instrument measures the underlying abstract concept (Nunnally, 1978). In this case, a researcher may assess the degree to which a measure adheres to standard definitions of depression such as that presented in agreed-upon diagnostic criteria (e.g. DSM-IV). Other forms of validity include criterion validity (also referred to as predictive or concurrent validity). This refers to how well the measure obtained from the instrument correlates with other measures of the same construct or some outcome that would be expected to correlate with the construct being assessed. This is typically measured by assessing the association of the measure with other self-rated or clinician-rated measures of depression. However, it may also be tested by examining correlations between scores on the instrument and measures of functional impairment.

Two of the most important features of good self-assessment instruments for depression are to be able to capture symptoms of depression and detect changes of depression with treatment (Cusin et al., 2009). The concept of depression has evolved over the past decades from depressive reaction (DSM-I, 1952), to depressive neurosis (DSM-II, 1968), and to major depressive disorder (MDD) (DSM-III, 1980; DSM-IV, 1994). The change in the conceptualization and definition of clinical depression over time necessitates the modification and revision of self-assessment instruments to accurately capture the symptoms of depression comprised by the most current definitions. In the next section, we will review the evolution of the concept of clinical depression, which has had significant impact on the development of self-assessment instruments for this disorder.

The evolution of the concept of major depressive disorder

In the earlier versions of the DSM (DSM-I and DSM-II), psychiatric diagnoses were based on a theoretical formulation of an assumed etiology, such as the development of neurosis as a result of unresolved early childhood experience. Psychiatric diagnoses in those versions were explained in narrative descriptions, which allowed much room for the clinician's personal interpretation and judgment. Due to the lack of an explicit definition of depression, instruments developed during that time had heterogeneous domains of depressive symptoms shaped by the various concepts of depression held by different researchers. It was not until 1980, with the publication of the DSM-III, that a significant change was adopted in how psychiatric disorders were diagnosed.

The DSM-III and the subsequent DSM-IV classifications depict psychiatric disorders as unique diagnostic entities defined by explicit diagnostic criteria generated by the consensus of leading psychiatric nosologists at the time.

Patients with a major depressive episode need to have five out of the nine stated depressive symptoms (depressed mood, loss of interest or pleasure, sleep disturbance, feelings of worthlessness or excessive or inappropriate guilt, fatigue, decreased concentration, change in appetite, psychomotor retardation or agitation, and suicidality), with at least one of the symptoms as either depressed mood or loss of interest or pleasure. The symptoms need to have been present for at least 2 weeks, represent a change from previous functioning, and have resulted in significant distress and/or functional impairment (DSM-III, 1980; DSM-IV, 1994). To be diagnosed with MDD, the symptoms and impairment from the major depressive episode cannot be better accounted for by other major psychotic disorders and the patient must not have had a manic episode at some point in his/her life. The use of a standardized concept of major depressive disorder (MDD), defined by explicit diagnostic criteria in DSM-III and DSM-IV, has revolutionized the task of instrument development for MDD (Murphy, 2002). It has led to the revision of instruments that were developed prior to DSM-III, such as the Beck Depression Inventory (BDI), and the development of new instruments based on the criteria defined in DSM-III and DSM-IV, including the Inventory of Depressive Symptomatology (IDS), the Quick Inventory of Depressive Symptomatology (QIDS), and the Patient Health Questionnaire-9 (PHQ-9). In the following section, we present descriptions of some of the most widely used and well-tested self-rated depression scales, as well as a review of their psychometric properties.

The Beck Depression Inventory (BDI, BDI-IA, and BDI-II)

The BDI, or Beck Depression Inventory, is a 21-question instrument developed by Aaron T. Beck in 1961 as a tool to evaluate depression in patients. At the time, physician diagnoses of depression were often inconsistent (Beck et al., 1961). Since its inception, the BDI has undergone two revisions, one in 1978 to the version known as the BDI-IA, and another in 1996 to the BDI-II. The BDI exists in a short form version as well.

The BDI consists of 21 questions based on 21 symptoms and attitudes, which clinical observation has attributed to be characteristics of depressed patients. These behavioral manifestations of depression are mood, pessimism, sense of failure, lack of satisfaction, feelings of guilt, sense of punishment, self-dislike, self-accusation, suicidal wishes, crying, irritability, social withdrawal, indecisiveness, distortion of body image, work inhibition, sleep disturbance, fatigability, loss of appetite, weight loss, somatic preoccupation, and loss of libido. The questions are rated on a scale of 0 to 3, in terms of symptom severity. Score cut-off ranges are generally defined as follows: minimal depression, < 10; mild to moderate depression, 10 to 18; moderate to severe depression, 19 to 29; and severe depression, 30 to 63. Beck has stressed that the score ranges are not absolute, and their interpretation should depend on both the population examined and the purpose of the evaluation. For example, in subclinical populations such as university students, the high total BDI scores may not be representative of depression, but of diffuse maladaptive functioning (Beck et al., 1988). Clinical trials employing differing standards and populations have been performed to determine the internal consistency of the BDI. The mean coefficient alpha of the BDI items was found to be 0.86 for psychiatric patients and 0.81 for non-psychiatric patients, showing high internal consistency of its items in both populations (Beck et al., 1988).

In 1978, the BDI underwent its first revision. Revisions included the removal or rewording of certain responses, as well as the removal of double-negatives. The time frame assessed was increased from how the patient "was feeling today," to how has the patient "been feeling for the past week, including today" (Beck et al., 1996). The internal consistency for both versions of the BDI was examined by a distribution of the original BDI to 598 inpatients and outpatients, and distribution of the BDI-IA to 248 outpatients. The coefficient alpha for the original BDI version was 0.88, and the coefficient alpha for the revised BDI-IA version was 0.86 (Beck & Steer, 1984). Although the BDI-IA and BDI were found to have high levels of internal consistency, many physicians continued to use the BDI because the existence of the BDI-IA was relatively poorly known.

The BDI was revised most recently in 1996 to the BDI-II to make its symptom and diagnostic criteria more reflective of the description for major depression described by the American Psychiatric Association's DSM-III-R/DSM-IV. The BDI-II remains composed of 21 symptoms, but 4 new symptoms were added and 4 discarded. The symptoms added were depression criteria included in the DSM-IV, but not addressed in the BDI-IA. The four new symptoms are agitation, worthlessness, concentration difficulty, and loss of energy. Four symptoms – weight loss, distortion of body image, work inhibition, and somatic preoccupation – were discarded because they were considered less indicative of the overall severity of depression. The BDI-II also addresses sleep and appetite increases. Finally, the time frame of depression was increased from how the patient has "been feeling for the past week, including today," to describe how the patient has been "feeling for the past two weeks, including today" (Steer et al., 1998). In a clinical study, the BDI-IA and the BDI-II were distributed to 140 psychiatric outpatients with varying psychiatric disorders for self-administration of the questionnaires. The coefficient alphas were 0.89 in regard to the BDI-IA and 0.91 for the BDI-II. These results are indicative of high internal consistencies (Beck et al., 1996).

The BDI has become one of the most widely used instruments for assessing the degree of depression in both the psychiatric patient population and in the normal population. Validities of the BDI were high with respect to the Hamilton Rating Scale for Depression (HRSD), and correlation with the two depression subscales of the Symptom Checklist-90R (SCL-90R) (Dozois, 2003). As stated in the studies above, the internal consistencies of the BDI, BDI-IA, and BDI-II have been demonstrated to be high as well. The BDI and BDI-II were tested on a sample of subjects which showed that BDI-II had improved clinical sensitivity, with reliability (alpha = 0.92) higher than that of the BDI (alpha = 0.86) (Beck et al., 1988; Steer et al., 1998). This is an indication of the success of its revision to become more up-to-date and user-friendly. While many of the self-assessment instruments (e.g. QIDS and CES-D) are available to the public free of charge, users of BDI-II are required to purchase the instrument. For those with limited resources, this could be a disincentive to use the BDI-II.

The Center for Epidemiological Studies Depression Scale (CES-D)

The Center for Epidemiological Studies Depression Scale (CES-D) was developed with support from the US National Institute of Mental Health (NIMH) (Radloff, 1977). It is a 20-item self-administered scale designed to measure depressive symptoms in the general (non-psychiatric) population. The scale asks for feelings and symptoms during the preceding week, and it measures the major components of depressive symptomatology, including depressive mood, feelings of guilt and worthlessness, psychomotor retardation, loss of appetite, and sleep disturbance.

Respondents indicate the frequency or duration of time in the past week that they experienced these symptoms and report the severity of the symptoms, which range from 0 to 3; 0 indicates that the symptoms occurred rarely or none of the time, 1 indicates some or a little of the time, 2 indicates occasionally or a moderate amount of time, and 3 indicates most or all of the time. Four items are worded in a positive direction to break tendencies towards response set, as well as to assess positive affect. The scale only takes a few minutes to score by hand. A total score for the scale is made by summing all items for each patient, except that the scores are reversed for the aforementioned four items. The total score has a range of 0 to 60.

In a validation study using data from five psychiatric populations and a community sample, Weissman et al. (1977) compared the CES-D with established self-report scales, including the Symptoms Checklist (SCL-90), the Hamilton Rating Scale for Depression (HRSD), the Raskin Depression Scale, and with ratings by experienced mental health workers. They found that CES-D had good agreement with other established self-report scales and with the clinicians' ratings. Using a cut-off score of 16 or above as the screening criterion for "caseness," the CES-D was found to be a sensitive tool for detecting depressive symptoms and change in symptoms over time in psychiatric populations.

In more recent studies, the CES-D was still found to be a reliable and valid instrument for identifying patients with depressive symptoms. Thomas et al. (2001) compared the CES-D with the Diagnostic Interview Schedule for the

DSM-IV in a population of low-income minority women at primary care clinics. They found that the standard cut-off score of ≥ 16 yielded a sensitivity of 0.95 and a specificity of 0.70 in predicting MDD, indicating that the CES-D appears to be valid for this demographic group. A few years later, Stahl et al. (2008) compared the CES-D against the DSM-IV–based Schedule for Clinical Assessment in Neuropsychiatry (SCAN) in a multiethnic population with diabetes in Singapore and found that the CES-D's cut-off score of 16 showed high negative predictive values of more than 90% in the population. This suggests that the CES-D is a reliable and valuable screening tool for clinical depression.

The CES-D has been used extensively because it is quick to administer, and it provides an indication that positive response should be investigated further. The limitations of CES-D is that it was designed before the publication of the DSM-III and thus does not assess the full range of depressive symptoms (e.g. suicidality) described in DSM-III and DSM-IV, and it also only assesses the occurrence of symptoms during the past week instead of the past 2 weeks, as stated in the required criteria of both DSM-III and DSM-IV.

The Inventory of Depressive Symptomatology (IDS-SR) and the Quick Inventory of Depressive Symptomatology (QIDS)

The IDS was designed to measure specific signs and symptoms of depression in both inpatients and outpatients. The Inventory of Depressive Symptomatology–Self- Report (IDS-SR) was originally developed in 1982 to address several limitations in existing self-reports for depression. Various standards for self-reports such as the BDI, the Zung Depression Scale, and the Carroll Rating Scale suffer from disadvantages such as unequal weighting to different symptoms and lack of certain endogenous symptoms. The original IDS-SR (IDS-SR$_{28}$) contains 28 items, all equally weighted and each rated from 0 to 3, where a higher rating indicates increasing severity. The items were clinically selected to include all symptoms required by DSM-III to diagnose a major depressive episode and melancholic symptom features, to include all symptoms used to define endogenous depression by Research Diagnostic Criteria, and to include items often used to differentiate patients with atypical, endogenous, and anxious depression. A 30-item version (IDS-SR$_{30}$) was also later developed to include all melancholic and atypical criterion symptoms for DSM-IV. A total of 26 of the 28 items (28 of 30 for the IDS-SR$_{30}$) contribute to the final score, since for both appetite and weight, only the increase or decrease in each is rated. Wording on the IDS-SR reflects the DSM focus on frequency, not the intensity of symptoms.

Rush's initial study (Rush et al., 1986) ($n = 289$) showed that the IDS-SR$_{28}$ had a high degree of internal consistency (coefficient alpha$|=|0.85$) and significantly correlated with both the Hamilton Rating Scale for Depression (HRSD; Pearson

$r = 0.67$) and the BDI (Pearson $r = 0.78$). Items such as lack of involvement, decreased concentration and decision making, sad mood, decreased energy, diminished capacity for pleasure, anxious mood, and future outlook correlated most highly with the total score. For concurrent validity, partial correlations between IDS-SR$_{28}$ and both BDI and HRSD individually were both higher than that between BDI and HRSD. As for construct validity, IDS-SR$_{28}$ scores for depressed subjects were significantly higher than for those with other diagnoses and normal controls ($p < 0.001$). The IDS-SR$_{28}$ was equivalent to the BDI and the HRSD in correctly classifying endogenous and non-endogenous patients.

A later study (Rush et al., 1996) demonstrated that both the IDS-SR$_{28}$ and IDS-SR$_{30}$ had internal consistency and concurrent validity and were able to differentiate between symptomatic and euthymic subjects ($p < 0.0001$). In addition, analysis of sensitivity to change in symptom severity in an open-label trial of fluoxetine ($n = 58$) showed that the IDS-SR$_{30}$ was highly related to the HRSD. The authors argued that the more complete atypical symptom feature coverage by the IDS-SR$_{30}$ makes it preferable to the IDS-SR$_{28}$ for research purposes.

The 16-item Quick Inventory of Depressive Symptomatology Self Report (QIDS-SR) was constructed in 2000 by selecting 16 items from IDS-SR$_{30}$ and converting these responses into 9 DSM-IV symptom criterion domains: sad mood, concentration, self-criticism, suicidal ideation, interest, energy/fatigue, sleep disturbance, decrease/increase in appetite/weight, and psychomotor agitation/retardation. In Rush's study looking at the QIDS-SR ($n = 596$), it had a high degree of internal consistency (coefficient alpha $= 0.86$), and its total scores were highly correlated with the IDS-SR$_{30}$ (0.96) and HRSD$_{17, 21, 24}$ (0.81–0.84) (Rush et al., 2003). In addition, QIDS-SR was as sensitive as the IDS-SR$_{30}$ in detecting change and defining response and remission.

The Patient Health Questionnaire-9 (PHQ-9)

The PHQ-9 is the depression module of the Patient Health Questionnaire (PHQ), a self-administered instrument for screening for common mental disorders in primary care. The nine items of the PHQ-9 assess each of the nine DSM-IV criteria on major depressive disorder, and patients rate each item as "0" (not at all) to "3" (nearly every day). As a severity measure, the PHQ-9 total score can range from 0 to 27. An item was also added to the end of the diagnostic portion of the PHQ-9 asking patients who checked off any problems on the questionnaire, "How *difficult* have these problems made it for you to do your work, take care of things at home, or get along with other people?" to assess degree of impairment.

In a validation study on PHQ-9, Kroenke et al. (2001) asked 6000 patients in 8 primary care clinics and 7 obstetrics-gynecology clinics to complete the screening instrument. The scores of the PHQ-9 in measuring the severity of depression were compared with those obtained from the 20-item Short-Form General Health Survey (SF-20) and correlated with self-reported sick days and clinic visits and symptom-related difficulty. Kroenke et al. reported that increase in PHQ-9 scores was related to decrease in functional status on all six SF-20 subscales and increased symptom-related difficulty, sick days, and health care utilization.

In the same study, the authors assessed the validity of the PHQ-9 as a screening instrument for depression by comparing it against an independently structured interview with a mental health professional as the criterion standard in a sub-sample of 580 patients. Using PHQ-9 score ≥ 10 as the cut-off for recognition of MDD, the self-assessment instrument had a sensitivity of 88% and a specificity of 88% for a major depressive episode. PHQ-9 scores of 5, 10, 15, and 20 repre-sented mild, moderate, moderately severe, and severe depression, respectively. Results were similar in the primary care and obstetrics-gynecology samples. The authors concluded that the PHQ-9 is also a reliable and valid measure of depression severity. These characteristics plus its brevity make the PHQ-9 a useful clinical and research tool for depression.

Internet-based self-assessment instruments for depression

Technological advances, including computerization of self-assessment and post-ing self-assessment instruments on the Internet, have tremendous potential for increasing patient and clinician access to self-assessment instruments. When the idea of using computers to assess psychiatric symptoms was first proposed, it was met with much skepticism. Recent studies have found that computer-ized assessments offer several advantages to clinical interviews. For example, such assessments are administered in an automated and standardized format, reduce the need for clinician time, provide increased reliability and consistency of administration, score data automatically, decrease errors due to scoring or data entry, and store data in a format that can be analyzed with statistical soft-ware (Butcher, 1987). In addition, some individuals find it easier to disclose sensitive information to a computer than to a clinician (Greist et al., 1974). Kobak et al. (1994) investigated subjects' satisfaction and reaction to computer- and clinician-administered versions of the HRSD and Hamilton Anxiety Scale among outpatients with and without psychiatric disorders and found that sub-jects' reactions to clinician- and computer-administered interviews were similar in the areas of overall comfort level and ease in answering questions. The sub-jects felt that clinicians were more sensitive to their needs and were better in determining how subjects felt and in asking questions specific to their feelings. On the other hand, subjects felt less embarrassed giving information to the computer.

With the recent explosion in the use of the Internet, self-assessment instruments can be made readily available online and will then be at the fingertips of people who want to use the self-assessment instruments. Powerful online search engines currently make computerized self-assessment instruments readily available to people who have Internet access and familiarity with Internet search options. Recently, there is growing interest in the use of the Internet as a tool for health services, including as a means for disseminating health education, searching for health providers, and delivering online treatment either by clinician using telecommunication or through automated programs (see Chapter 4 on self-help interventions for a complete review of such programs). Web-based screening instruments for depression and anxiety disorders have been developed and tested and were found to be acceptable and reliable depression screening tools (Farvolder et al., 2003; Lin et al., 2007).

Houston et al. (2001) investigated the use and the performance of an Internet-based depression screening tool. They placed a computerized CES-D on a large online health information portal owned by Aetna US Healthcare. During an 8-month period, the CES-D scale was completed 24,479 times, and 58% screened positive for depression. They concluded that the Internet provides a continuously available, inexpensive, easily maintained platform to anonymously screen a large number of individuals from a broad geographic area. However, they did find the limitation that older adults and minorities may visit the screening sites less frequently than other populations. This program is exemplary in its use of a previously validated instrument as the basis for self-assessment online. Unfortunately, some depression self-assessments that users find through search engines may be untested and of dubious origin. In Tabel 4.1, we provide a patient hand-out that lists websites where patients can access several valid depression assessment instruments at no cost.

The application of self-assessment instruments

Thus far, self-assessment instruments are under-utilized both in research and in clinical practice. Self-assessment instruments have much potential to be used in monitoring depression severity in both research and clinical practice, for quality improvement in institutions, and for self-management.

Monitoring clinical outcomes

As we have discussed earlier in the chapter, self-assessment instruments are easy to administer, and there is increasing evidence to show the validity of well-designed instruments in measuring severity of depression as defined by the DSM-IV, the latest version of the diagnostic manual of psychiatric disorders. The recent endorsement by the FDA of the use of the self-rated versions of the IDS and QIDS to measure depression outcomes in clinical trials supports the trend. The use of self-assessment instruments will be increasingly employed in clinical trials since it is inexpensive to use, and online self-assessment instruments allow symptom monitoring without the limits of geographical barriers. This new approach in data collection could revolutionize the design and execution of clinical trials. Similar changes may also take place in clinical practice. Routine use of self-assessment instruments allows systematic and continuous monitoring of patients' depression symptoms to gauge patients' treatment response and to detect relapse of depression at an early stage. In addition, the use of self-reporting of severity of symptoms may help patients to have a more objective appraisal of their clinical condition.

Quality improvement

Self-assessment instruments for depression can also be used for quality improvement of clinical services. In the past decades, there has been an increasing awareness among clinics, community health centers, hospitals, and health insurance companies of the need to monitor the outcomes of clinical services. Data are usually collected longitudinally by these institutions so that the outcomes of treatment of depression can be compared over time and among different institutions. Based on the information collected, leaders in different institutions may design, implement, and evaluate the usefulness of their quality improvement measures to improve the quality of clinical services. The aforementioned self-assessment instruments are useful tools to monitor the outcomes of depression treatments.

There has been a growing group of organizations which advocate rewarding high-quality clinical services using a pay-for-performance approach to quality improvement (Rosenthal, 2008). The Institute of Medicine (IOM) has recommended that Medicare should gradually replace its current fee-for-service payment system with a new pay-for-performance system for reimbursing participating health care providers (IOM, 2006). The use of self-assessment instruments to measure treatment outcomes of depression in different institutions could serve as one of the indices of clinical improvement.

Self-management of depression

A growing area in the use of self-assessment instruments is for self-management of depression, the core theme of this book. As noted previously, individuals may use self-assessment instruments to self-recognize the severity of their depression in the course of treatment. People with remitted depression could also use the instruments to detect whether depression has relapsed, as symptoms of depression tend to fluctuate over time. Patients can use self-assessment to identify how psychosocial stressors and coping efforts affect the severity of their depression. Based on this feedback, patients may calibrate their use of self-management strategies accordingly. In addition, self-assessment instruments have tremendous potential as a tool for depression self-screening, which will be described in greater detail in the second half of this chapter. As self-assessment instruments are becoming increasingly available online, they may become an integral part of health care in the near future.

Limitations of self-assessment instruments for measuring severity of depression

While self-assessment instruments are standardized, reliable, and are relatively inexpensive to use, their accuracy in measuring severity of depression is contingent upon the presence of a host of factors, which include the following: the items of the instruments are clear, easy to understand, and adequately measure the intended concept; the patients are able to recognize their symptoms and are able to describe them correctly; and the patients are motivated and able to concentrate to accurately report their symptoms.

Most self-assessment instruments are developed using a small number of relatively homogeneous populations, and they may not be accurate when they are used to measure depression in subjects who come from different age groups, severity levels, levels of education, and cultural backgrounds. Self-assessment instruments have the advantage of not being biased by clinicians' judgment, which could be subjective and not reliable. However, these self-reports do not provide any information on whether the subjects are awake, alert, and have the cognitive ability to report accurately, or have the tendency of under- or over-reporting their symptoms. These instruments also do not inform whether the reported symptoms were due to depression or due to other comorbid medical and/or psychiatric disorders. Finally, the most important question is: Will self-assessment instruments be utilized by patients, and if so, will patients receive better treatment for their depression? These remaining questions lead to the discussion later in this chapter of the complementary role of clinicians in using and interpreting the results of self-assessment instruments.

Self-assessment instruments for depression screening

As discussed in our earlier chapters, depression is a common disorder which could become debilitating if left untreated. It is estimated that 5% to 12% of men and 10% to 25% of women have a major depressive episode during their lifetime (Kessler et al., 1994). If left untreated, depressive disorders are associated with functional impairment, decreased productivity, increased health care utilization, and increased risk for suicide. Instead of directly seeking help from mental health professionals, most patients with depression are treated in the primary care setting. Unfortunately, 35% to 70% of primary care patients with depression are not diagnosed or receive inadequate treatment (Tiemens et al., 1996; Hirschfeld et al., 1997). Active depression screening has been proposed as a way to improve recognition of depression in primary care. To improve recognition of MDD, the US Preventive Services Task Force (USPSTF, 2002) has recommended routine screening for depression in "primary care settings that have systems in place to assure accurate diagnosis, effective treatment, and follow-up." Compared with clinician interview and clinician-rated screenings, self-assessment instruments are much more cost-effective ways of depression screening.

There is extensive literature on the development and validation of the use of various self-assessment instruments for depression screening. We will review the methodology involved and the characteristics of common instruments for depression screening. We will also look at the effectiveness and cost-effectiveness of depression screening using self-assessment instruments, including web-based assessments.

Selecting a cut-off score for "caseness" for a screening instrument

Self-assessment scales are quantitative, dimensional measurement of symptoms of depression. In using self-assessment scales to screen for patients with depression, it requires categorizing people into those who are "case" (i.e. depression severity is clinically significant) and those who are "non-case" (i.e. depression symptoms severity is below clinical threshold). This is usually done by (1) summing up the items of the scale to generate a total score, and (2) selecting a threshold or "cut-off score." People who score at or above the threshold of the screening scale are considered "positive screens" or "cases," and those who score below the threshold are "negative screens" or "non-cases." For example, patients who score 10 or above on the PHQ-9 scale have "screened positive," while patients who score 9 less or less on the PHQ-9 have "screened negative" (Kroenke et al., 2001).

Such an approach fits into the medical model which involves diagnosing the presence of a disorder in order to form the basis for treatment. However, it may appear that such a categorization is an arbitrary one. For a scale to be a good instrument for depression screening, the items of the scale need to map correctly to the concept and symptoms of depression, with appropriate weighting of its items so that the total score of the scale accurately reflects the severity of depression. In the next section, we will discuss how to determine the validity of a self-assessment instrument as a tool for depression screening.

The validity of a self-assessment instrument for depression screening

Investigating the validity of a screening scale requires comparison of the results of said screening instrument with the results of a "gold standard." In the absence of objective laboratory tests for psychiatric disorders, researchers have used the diagnoses obtained by expert clinicians using standardized instruments as the gold standard (criterion instruments). The validity of a screening instrument is generally expressed by its sensitivity, specificity, positive predictive power, and negative predictive power. Sensitivity is a measure of the screening instrument's ability to detect the true cases of a disorder identified by the criterion instrument. Specificity is a measure of the screening instrument's ability to identify the true non-cases identified by the criterion instrument. Higher values of sensitivity and specificity are always desirable. Positive predictive power is the proportion of apparent cases, as detected by the screening instrument, that are true cases as determined by the criterion instrument. Negative predictive power is the proportion of apparent non-cases, as detected by the screening instrument, that are true non-cases as determined by the criterion instrument. For a given screening instrument, higher sensitivity is obtained by lowering the cut-off score for caseness, which in turn will lower the specificity and vice versa. The only way to improve both sensitivity and specificity without such a trade-off is to improve the diagnostic accuracy of the instrument itself.

Commonly used self-assessment instruments for depression screening

The commonly used self-assessment instruments described earlier in this chapter have all been validated for use as depression screening instruments. Instead of using a single cut-off score to categorize subjects into "case" and "non-case," many of these instruments use multiple cut-off scores to categorize people into different levels of severity of their depression. For the CES-D, the score of 15 was selected to be the cut-off score: people with CES-D scores of 15 to 21 are considered mild to moderately depressed, and people with CES-D scores > 21 are considered as having a high possibility of having clinical depression (Radloff, 1977). For the PHQ-9, the scores of 9 or below are considered asymptomatic; 10 to 14, mildly depressed; 15 to 19, moderately depressed; and > 19, severely depressed (Kroenke et al., 2001). For BDI-II, scores of 0 to 13 are considered minimal depression, 14 to 19, mild depression; 20 to 28, moderate depression; and 29 to 63, severe depression (Beck et al., 1996). With the QIDS-SR, scores of 6 to 10 are considered mildly depressed; 11 to 15, moderately depressed; 16 to 20, severely depressed; and > 21, very severely depressed (http://www.ids-qids.org/). These proposed cut-off points and the interpretation of the scores of the scales are adopted from sources listed in Table 2.1.

With recent advancement in technology, many of the above self-assessment instruments are available. Anyone with access to the Internet can easily obtain a copy of the instrument. Even more importantly, researchers can now use the Internet as a continuously available, inexpensive, easily maintained platform to screen a large number of individuals from a broad geographic area. In the Houston et al. (2001) study described earlier, the researchers investigated using the Internet-based CES-D for screening the public for depression by placing it within a large online health information portal owned by Aetna US Healthcare. Within the 8-month study period, the CES-D scale was completed 24,479 times, at a reasonably low cost of $12,750. In this study, subjects remained anonymous, a highly desirable feature for those who worry about being identified and labeled as having depression. In the same study, patients received feedback based on the probability of their having depression: those who scored in the moderate range were instructed to seek further advice from a health professional or to return later and retake the test. Participants who scored above 22 were told that they had a high likelihood of clinical depression and were advised to seek treatment from a health professional. Although the study did not have a follow-up component to assess the effectiveness of the program, it illustrated the feasibility and the potential usefulness of online depression screening.

Limitations of depression screening using self-assessment instruments

The goal of depression screening is to improve recognition and treatment of depression, particularly for people with unrecognized depression. Yet it is unclear whether improved recognition of depression leads to actual treatment of depression and to improved outcomes of depression symptoms.

In 1980, Linn and Yager randomized 150 new patients in an ambulatory care setting into three groups; group 1 was screened for depression and results were given to primary care physicians (PCPs) before the visits, group 2 was screened for depression and results were given to PCPs after the visits, and group 3 received no depression screening. Later they investigated the outcomes by reviewing the medical records of the subjects. They found that 42% of the 100 patients screened with the Zung self-rating depression scale had scores outside the normal range. Chart notation about depression was effectively and appropriately increased by feedback and sensitization from 8% to 25%, but only 12% of the entire sample received any type of treatment for depression.

In a study in a primary care setting in the UK, Dowrick and Buchan (1995) used BDI for depression screening and identified 116 patients with undetected depression. Forty-five percent of the identified subjects were randomly chosen to have their BDI disclosed to the general practitioners. Dowrick and Buchan found that the rate of diagnosis was higher in the disclosed group, but intent to treat was only marginally higher. In another study, Whooley et al. (2000)

screened elderly primary care patients for depression using the Geriatric Depression Scale (GDS) in 13 primary care clinics randomized into intervention clinic and non-intervention clinics. PCPs in intervention clinics were notified of their patients' GDS scores with treatment recommendations, and participants in the intervention clinics with GDS scores suggestive of depression were offered educational group sessions. Participants were followed for 2 years and no benefit in improvement in depression severity was found from case-finding and intensive patient education.

Gilbody et al. (2005) reviewed 12 studies and investigated the clinical use and cost-effectiveness of screening and case finding instruments. They concluded that routine screening and feedback of depression have no impact on the detection of depression, management, or outcome of depression. However, this conclusion must be qualified in that studies using a collaborative care approach were not included in this review, since they include many active components and the reviewers felt that it would be difficult to disentangle the effectiveness of screening from other components.

These studies point out that depression screening, when conducted in isolation, has limited impact on the treatment of depression. This reinforces the importance of redesigning the structure of primary care services to implement the Collaborative Care Model: to coordinate the services provided by primary care physicians, specialists, and care managers, and by tapping into community resources to better treat chronic illnesses (Wagner, 1998). As we described in Chapter 1, our approach to self-management is informed by the Collaborative Care Model which involves multidisciplinary team members: PCPs, care managers, and specialists. Such a model acknowledges that self-assessment (including screening) is likely most effective in the context of other intervention strategies that we discuss in detail in subsequent chapters.

Role of clinicians in the use of self-assessment instruments

Until now, self-assessment instruments have been predominantly used in clinical studies, and they are under-utilized in clinical practices and as self-management tools. There is ample opportunity for clinicians to extend the use of these instruments to improve treatment and recognition of depression.

Monitoring severity of depression

Clinicians should advocate the use of these instruments as a means to obtain frequent, inexpensive measurements of the severity of depression. They may also provide patients with these instruments, educate them on the usefulness of these instruments for self-management of depression, or instruct them to download the instruments from the Internet. However, simply making these self-assessment instruments available is not sufficient. Clinicians should make it routine during each clinical visit for patients to report the severity of their symptoms based on the instruments, similar to the routine measurement of body temperature and blood pressure in medical visits. In addition, clinicians should try to integrate data from self-assessment instruments with their understanding of the patient's personal, psychosocial, medical, and psychiatric history to determine the best treatment for the patient in concordance with the patient's illness beliefs and preferences.

Depression screening

Primary care physicians need to understand their role in taking care of the overall well-being of their patients and not to consider mental illnesses less important or not part of their responsibilities. While medical professionals may focus their practice in specialized areas in medicine or on certain illnesses, most patients continue to view primary care physicians as gate-keepers for their medical and mental problems. If primary care physicians acknowledge such a role, they should take the lead in adopting depression screening to decrease unrecognized depression. They may use instruments ranging from a paper and pencil questionnaire to specific websites to perform depression screening, engage patients identified with depression in treatment, and involve mental health professionals and other community resources when needed.

Screening for depression can also be considered in medical inpatient settings and in community settings such as nursing homes, where the prevalence of depression is high and resources for mental health expertise are limited. Some mental health clinicians routinely ask all new patients to complete a depression assessment regardless of presenting problem. In addition to screening for the possible presence of depression, it can be especially helpful as a non-intrusive method of gauging suicide risk. In addition, in cases where depression is a focus of treatment, this initial score can then be used as a baseline assessment of symptoms for comparison with later assessments after treatments have been initiated.

Practical considerations: how to adopt self-assessment instruments in your practice

To adopt the use of self-assessment instruments, clinicians may start by selecting a measure and be prepared to spend time to educate their patients about the benefits of using the instruments, tracking the measurements during follow-up visits, and integrating patients' self-assessment into their treatment plans.

(a) *Selecting a measure.* All the instruments described in the chapter have good psychometric qualities and are widely used in research. To select among these options, one may consider the goal of self-assessment, whether it is for monitoring clinical outcomes or for mass depression screening. For the latter, The PHQ-9 could be a practical choice, as it is a brief instrument designed and validated for depression screening in primary care settings. Other factors to consider may include the length and the scope of symptoms measured by the instrument, whether the wordings of the instrument are easily understandable, the ease of scoring the items, and the costs involved. For instance, CES-D does not assess suicidality, and that is a significant limitation, in our opinion. In some large-scale screening for research purposes, this may be desirable from a liability perspective, as it is not always feasible to follow up promptly upon this information. However, in the context of an established clinical relationship, screening of suicidality is highly valuable, especially in light of concerns about possible increased suicidality associated with some pharmacological treatments. Also, different measures may highlight different aspects of depression. For instance, the BDI-II provides greater focus on cognitive components of depression, such as attitudes of pessimism and personal shortcomings. A more detailed assessment of cognition may be more relevant for treatment approaches such as cognitive behavioral therapy (CBT) and other forms of psychotherapy. The IDS-SR$_{30}$ includes a complete list of typical and atypical depression symptoms, and thus it may be a better choice for monitoring response to pharmacotherapy. The BDI-II has revised the wordings from the BDI version and has become a more user-friendly instrument. Yet users of the BDI-II are required to purchase the instrument, making it less favorable compared with CES-D and QIDS-SR, which are in the public domain.

(b) *Explaining to patients the importance of using self-assessment instruments.* It is important to explain to patients the benefits of self-assessment so that they are willing to spend the time and efforts in accurately reporting their symptoms. For instance, clinicians may explain that self-assessment is a good way to check if treatment is helping and to monitor symptoms to make sure we detect any worsening as early as possible. Although filling out the questionnaire takes a bit of time, it helps to understand how the patients are doing in between visits. In addition, it provides a systematic review of patients' symptoms before visits to allow the clinician to spend more time to discuss treatment options with patients. By using the self-assessment instruments, patients may have an accurate understanding of what depression is: Patients aren't always aware of the range of symptoms involved in the syndrome of depression. Repeatedly completing assessments helps to solidify their understanding of the concept. In addition, self-monitoring facilitates insight into the connection between self-help efforts and improvement. For instance, as a patient reviews periods when symptoms are relatively lower or higher, they can think about what actions they have taken that may have contributed to improvements (e.g. "my scores started to improve when I began exercising regularly").

(c) *Tracking the measurements over time.* It is frequently helpful to ask patients to chart their symptoms scores on a semi-regular basis, either manually, in a computer spreadsheet program, or through a computerized self-help program. Monitoring symptoms over time allows for a more accurate sense of the course of depression and of the impact of specific treatments on depressive symptoms. After an initial setback, a patient with depression may conclude "This treatment isn't working. I am doomed to always be depressed." However, reviewing symptom levels over the course of treatment can provide data that may challenge this overly pessimistic conclusion.

(d) *Integrating self-assessment into your clinical work.* This can be accomplished using low-tech approaches, which include having patients complete the instrument on paper before the visit. As such, you can have blank copies in the waiting room provided by a receptionist or in a self-service area. We have found that once patients are accustomed to this practice, it becomes a routine part of the visit. Alternatively, patients can be given access to the questionnaire online or given a blank copy to photocopy at home so that they can fill out the questionnaire before visits and bring it to each session or periodically (e.g. first session of the month if treatment sessions are held weekly). For patients who are familiar with computer use, they may submit data of their self-assessment electronically in-between appointments. This is particularly useful for patients with stable conditions who pay infrequent visits to their clinicians. In order to integrate self-assessment into clinical work, the clinicians need to review the measurements each time with patients and to plan treatment utilizing the information from self-assessment instruments.

Summary and conclusion

Self-rated and clinician-rated assessment instruments are the fundamental tools to collect reliable measurement for severity of depression and for mass depression screening. The explicit diagnostic criteria brought by the DSM-III and DSM-IV facilitate the development and use of standardized self-assessment instruments. There is growing evidence on the usefulness and validity of well-designed self-assessment instruments as measurement tools. The availability of information online has provided easy access to these self-assessment instruments, which are expected to become increasingly important in the recognition and treatment of depression, both for clinical practice and for research purposes.

REFERENCES

American Psychiatric Association. *Diagnostic and Statistical Manual of Mental Disorders.* 1st edn. Washington, DC: American Psychiatric Association; 1952.

American Psychiatric Association. *Diagnostic and Statistical Manual of Mental Disorders.* 2nd edn. Washington, DC: American Psychiatric Association; 1968.

American Psychiatric Association. *Diagnostic and Statistical Manual of Mental Disorders.* 3rd edn. Washington, DC: American Psychiatric Association; 1980.

American Psychiatric Association. *Diagnostic and Statistical Manual of Mental Disorders.* 4th edn. Washington, DC: American Psychiatric Assocation; 1994.

Beck AT, Steer RA. Internal consistencies of the original and revised Beck Depression Inventory. *J Clin Psych.* 1984; 40(6):1365–1367.

Beck AT, Ward CH, Mendelson M, Mock J. An inventory for measuring depression. *Erbaugh J Arch Gen Psych.* 1961; 4:561–571.

Beck AT, Steer RA, Garbin MG. Psychometric properties of the Beck Depression Inventory: twenty-five years of evaluation. *Clin Psych Rev.* 1988; 8:77–100.

Beck AT, Steer RA, Ball R, Ranieri WF. Comparison of Beck Depression Inventories–IA and –II in psychiatric outpatients. *J Pers Assess.* 1996; 67(3):588–597.

Beck AT, Steer RA, Brown GK. *BDI-II Manual.* San Antonio, TX: The Psychological Corporation/Harcourt Brace & Company; 1996, p 11.

Butcher JN. The use of computers in psychological assessment: an overview of practices and issues. In Butcher JN, ed: *Computerized Psychological Assessment.* New York: Basic Books; 1987, pp 3–14.

Cusin C, Yang H, Fava M. How to choose a primary efficacy measure in depression clinical trials: a primer for the clinical researcher. In Baer L and Blais M, eds: *Handbook of Clinical Rating Scales and Assessment and Psychiatry and Mental Health: Current Clinical Psychiatry.* New York: Springer Verlag; 2009.

Dowrick C, Buchan L. Twelve month outcome of depression in general practice: does detection or disclosure make a difference? *BMJ.* 1995; 311:1274–1276.

Dozois DJ. The psychometric characteristics of the Hamilton Depression Inventory. *J Pers Assess.* 2003; 80(1):31–40.

Farvolder P, McBride C, Bagby RM, Ravitz P. A web-based screening instrument for depression and anxiety disorders in primary care. *J Med Internet Res.* 2003; 5(3):e23.

Gilbody S, House AO, Sheldon TA. Screening and case finding instruments for depression. *Cochrane Database Syst Rev.* 2005; 19(4):CD002792.

Greist JH, Gustafson DH, Stauss FF, Rowse GL, Laughren TP, Chiles JA. Suicide risk prediction: a new approach. *Life Threat Behav.* 1974; 4:212–223.

Hirschfeld RM, Keller MB, Panico S, Arons BS, Barlow D, Davidoff F, Endicott J, Froom J, Goldstein M, Gorman JM, Marek RJ, Maurer TA, Meyer R, Phillips K, Ross J, Schwenk TL, Sharfstein SS, Thase ME, Wyatt RJ. The National Depressive and Manic-Depressive Association consensus statement on the undertreatment of depression. *JAMA.* 1997; 277(4):333–340.

Houston TK, Cooper LA, Vu HT, Kahn J, Toser J, Ford DE. Screening the public for depression through the internet. *Psych Serv.* 2001; 52(3):362–367.

Institute of Medicine (IOM). *Rewarding Provider Performance: Aligning Incentives in Medicare.* Washington, DC: National Academies Press; 2006.

Kessler RC, McGonagle KA, Zhao S, Nelson CB, Hughes M, Eshleman S, Wittchen HU, Kendler KS. Lifetime and 12-month prevalence of DSM-III-R psychiatric disorders in the United States. Results from the National Comorbidity Survey. *Arch Gen Psychiatry.* 1994; 51(1):8–19.

Kobak KA, Reynolds WM, Griest JH. Computerized and clinician assessment of depression and anxiety: respondent evaluation and satisfaction. *J Pers Assess.* 1994; 63(1):173–180.

Kroenke K, Spitzer RL, Williams JB. The PHQ-9: validity of a brief depression severity measure. *J Gen Intern Med.* 2001; 16(9):606–613.

Lin CC, Bai YM, Liu CY, Hsiao MC, Chen JY, Tsai SJ, Ouyang WC, Wu CH, Li YC. Web-based tools can be used reliably to detect patients with depressive disorder and subsyndromal depressive symptoms. *BMC Psychiatry.* 2007; 7(12):1–9.

Linn LS, Yager J. The effect of screening, sensitization, and feedback on notation of depression. *J Med Educ.* 1980; 55(11):942–949.

Murphy JM. Symptom scales and diagnostic schedules in adult psychiatry. In Tsuang MT, Tohen M, eds: *Textbook in Psychiatric Epidemiology.* 2nd edn. New York: Wiley; 2002, pp 273–332.

Nunnally JC. *Psychometric theory.* 2nd edn. New York: McGraw-Hill Book Company; 1978.

Radloff LS. The CES-D scale: a self-report depression scale for research in the general population. *Applied Psychol Measurement.* 1977; 1:385–401.

Rosenthal MB. Beyond pay for performance: merging models of provider payment reform. *N Engl J Med.* 2008; 359(12):1197–1200.

Rush AJ, Giles DE, Schlesser MA, Fulton CL, Weissenburger J, Burns C. The Inventory for Depressive Symptomatology (IDS): preliminary findings. *Psychiatry Res.* 1986; 18:65–87.

Rush AJ, Gullion CM, Basco MR, Jarrett RB, Trivedi MH. The Inventory of Depressive Symptomatology (IDS): psychometric properties. *Psychol Med.* 1996; 26:477–486.

Rush AJ, Trivedi MH, Ibrahim HM, Carmody TJ, Arnow B, Klein DN, Markowitz JC, Ninan PT, Kornstein S, Manber R, Thase ME, Kocsis JH, Keller MB. The 16-Item Quick Inventory of Depressive Symptomatology (QIDS), clinician rating (QIDS-C), and self-report (QIDS-SR): a psychometric evaluation in patients with chronic major depression. *Biol Psychiatry.* 2003; 54:573–583.

Stahl D, Sum CF, Lum SS, Liow PH, Chan YH, Verma S, Chua HC, Chong SA. Screening for depressive symptoms: validation of the Center for Epidemiologic Studies Depression scale (CES-D) in a multiethnic group of patients with diabetes in Singapore. *Diabetes Care.* 2008; 31(6):1118–1119.

Steer RA, Clark DA, Beck AT, Ranieri WF. Common and specific dimensions of self-reported anxiety and depression: the BDI-II versus the BDI-IA. *Behav Res Ther.* 1998; 37:183–190.

Thomas JL, Jones GN, Scarinci IC, Mehan DJ, Brantley PJ. The utility of the CES-D as a depression screening measure among low-income women attending primary care clinics. The Center for Epidemiologic Studies-Depression. *Int J Psychiatry Med.* 2001; 31(1):25–40.

Tiemens BG, Ormel J, Simon GE. Occurrence, recognition, and outcome of psychological disorders in primary care. *Am J Psychiatry.* 1996; 153(5):636–644.

United States Preventive Services Task Force. Depression Screening. May 2002. Available at http://www.ahrq.gov/clinic/uspstf/uspsdepr.htm

Wagner EH. Chronic disease management: what will it take to improve care for chronic illness? *Eff Clin Pract.* 1:2–4, 1998.

Wagner EH, Simon GE. Managing depression in primary care. *BMJ.* 2001; 322(7289):746–747.

Weissman MM, Sholomskas D, Pottenger M, Prusoff BA, Locke BZ. Assessing depressive symptoms in five psychiatric populations: a validation study. *Am J Epidemiol.* 1977; 106(3):203–214.

Whooley MA, Stone B, Soghikian K. Randomized trial of case-finding for depression in elderly primary care patients. *J Gen Intern Med.* 2000; 15(5):293–300.

Self-help

The role of bibliotherapy and computerized psychotherapy in self-management for depression

Self-help for depression and other psychiatric disorders is widely available. It is estimated that 2000 new self-help books are published each year (Rosen, 1993). Eighty percent of Internet users have sought health care information online, with mental health and relationship problems being among the most common search topics (Pew Internet and American Life Project, 2003). Between January and March of 2003, over 2 million Internet users worldwide conducted searches for information on depression (Lamberg, 2003). Self-help information and resources are available, and many people make use of them.

A growing body of research suggests that self-help delivered via books (i.e. bibliotherapy) and computer programs (i.e. computerized psychotherapy) may be efficacious in treating depression. However, these findings are restricted to specific self-help books and computer programs that have been formally tested. Indeed, some books and websites may contain inaccurate and potentially harmful information (Ernst & Schmidt, 2004; Griffiths & Christensen, 2000; Redding et al., in press). Thus it is important that clinicians know which resources have empirical support.

Although the term "self-help" implies a patient working entirely independent of any professional help, most successful self-help programs involve at least minimal clinician involvement. As such, book- or computer-based self-help can be easily integrated into a clinicians' plan for supporting a patient in self-managing depression. Indeed, as many as 85% of clinicians surveyed report recommending self-help books to at least one of their clients (Norcross, 2000).

In this chapter, we will first define bibliotherapy and computerized psychotherapy and discuss their relevance for self-management of depression. As with other chapters, we will critically review the research to assess the feasibility and efficacy of these approaches to the self-management of depression. We will then discuss the promises and challenges inherent in implementing bibliotherapy and computerized psychotherapy. Finally, we will present four models for integrating computerized psychotherapy into the treatment of depression in primary care and mental health care settings.

Definitions of bibliotherapy and computerized psychotherapy

Bibliotherapy is typically defined as the use of written texts as a means of personal development or alleviating distress (den Boer et al., 2004; Gregory et al., 2004; Marrs, 1995). Some definitions also include computer programs as a form of bibliotherapy, but for the sake of this review, bibliotherapy will be restricted to studies of printed materials. In bibliotherapy for depression, texts typically include information about depression and strategies for coping with it. The intervention is self-administered in that participants read and apply materials on their own time; however, bibliotherapy programs may also involve minimal contact with a clinician or participation in group sessions led by a professional facilitator, paraprofessional, or other patients.

It is also helpful to clarify approaches not included in this definition. Across time and cultures, reading great works of literature (e.g. poetry, fiction, memoirs) has been revered as a means to enhance personal development and can even be "therapeutic." Indeed, some psychotherapists will recommend to clients books or films depicting fictional or non-fictional accounts of people coping with mental illness or other adversity to stimulate a client's own processing of their own experience (Norcross, 2006). However, such approaches have received very little empirical study and thus will not be a focus here.

Computerized psychotherapy is a standardized, automated intervention delivered by a computer program to a user who accesses the program through software on a personal computer or from a distance via the Internet or the telephone. Such programs can be used to present patients and their families with information about depression and its treatment, which we will refer to as psychoeducation. These programs can also be used to teach strategies for managing depression. To date, the content of programs includes cognitive behavioral therapy (CBT) interventions. Programs can also be used to administer questionnaires to facilitate self-monitoring of symptoms. As we will note, such programs can be used as stand-alone interventions; however, they are typically more effective when there is at least minimal interaction with a live clinician.

For the sake of this review, we will not discuss online counseling, in which a clinician provides traditional psychotherapy over an electronic medium such as email or instant messaging. This approach has received little research attention as a treatment for depression. Furthermore, this approach is not consistent with self-management in that it still relies heavily on a clinician directing or facilitating care. This chapter will also not address online support groups, which will be discussed along with other peer-led support groups in Chapter 7. The majority of this review will focus on discussing computerized psychotherapy programs that have been tested in published, peer-reviewed research. However, given the rapidly evolving nature of this technology, we will also discuss some innovative and promising new computerized psychotherapy programs that are currently being developed and tested to give readers a sense of where this field is headed.

Bibliotherapy and computerized psychotherapy in the self-management of depression

Bibliotherapy and computerized psychotherapy are consistent with several of the objectives of self-management. Both approaches can be used to give patients more knowledge about their disorder and to self-monitor symptoms. Consistent with the importance of empowering patients and enhancing their self-efficacy, use of self-help materials can support patients' sense of responsibility in treatment and sense of control over their condition (Mains & Scogin, 2003). It is treatment that can be partially or fully self-administered, thereby reducing reliance on a clinician. Books and computerized psychotherapy programs also provide durable self-management skills that patients can continue to use beyond acute treatment for relapse prevention. With many programs, patients can access psychotherapy at a time of day convenient to their schedule and at a location of their choice. They can work at their own pace and review material often.

Computerized psychotherapy offers several additional advantages over bibliotherapy. Computerized programs are interactive; they can provide instant scores on symptom assessments and provide feedback on patients' responses to skill-building exercises. They can increase engagement through the use of audio and video, which may be especially relevant given the impairment in concentration that is characteristic of depression. Unlike books, Internet-based programs can be modified and updated on a large scale to keep up with new developments in clinical practice.

For patients with limited computer literacy or access to a computer or Internet, bibliotherapy may be a more comfortable fit than computerized psychotherapy. However, many patients may be more inclined to receive mental health services from a computer than one might estimate. As noted previously, many people seek out information on mental health and relationship problems on the Internet (Pew Internet and American Life Project, 2003; Sirovatka, 2002). A recent British survey of potential psychotherapy self-help users found that 91% wanted access to self-help via the Internet (Graham et al., 2001), and patients may prefer computer-based therapies to bibliotherapy as a self-help method for depression (Whitfield et al., 2005). There is also anecdotal evidence that some patients report feeling more comfortable disclosing some information to a computer rather than a therapist in a face-to-face encounter (Gega et al., 2004).

There are also many public policy advantages for bibliotherapy and computerized psychotherapy, either when used alone or in the context of a clinician-guided self-management program. Both have the potential of reducing therapist time per patient, thereby reducing the cost of mental health care. Both have the potential to present service to patients on psychotherapy waitlists where their condition may deteriorate. Both can reduce geographical- and transportation-related barriers to treatment. Other potential arguments for self-help are that patients can receive treatment anonymously, thereby reducing the stigma of seeking services. Primary care patients generally prefer psychotherapy to medication (e.g. Gum et al., 2006); however, medication is the most common first-line treatment for depression, in part because it is easily dispensed through primary care. However, self-help is potentially as easily exportable as medication and thus could give patients more choice in selecting their first-line treatment.

Research on bibliotherapy as a treatment for depression

Based upon the results of several meta-analyses, the effects of bibliotherapy on depression symptoms can be considered medium to large in magnitude relative to inactive control conditions (Cuijpers, 1997; Cuijpers, 1998; Gregory et al., 2004). The size of this effect is generally comparable to therapist-delivered cognitive behavioral therapy (CBT) for depression (den Boer et al., 2004). In studies where bibliotherapy was compared with a brief, therapist-delivered treatment for depression and anxiety, bibliotherapy performed nearly as well on average (den Boer et al., 2004). As noted previously, bibliotherapy studies typically involve some minimal contact with a researcher for assessments, reminders, or clarification of bibliotherapy material. In some cases, individuals read materials on their own and meet in a group with a therapist facilitator to discuss the reading. However, it should be noted that in the largest meta-analysis to date, no difference was found between the bibliotherapy programs that are individually administered and those that include a group meeting (Gregory et al., 2004).

As noted previously, not all self-help books are created equal. It is the small minority that has been tested empirically. Indeed, just because a book is based on an empirically supported treatment approach does not mean it will be effective as largely self-administered treatment (Rosen, 1987). Popularity of a book in terms of high sales is also not a guarantee of its validity. In a recent review of the 50 top-selling self-help books for depression, anxiety, and trauma, a group of researchers determined that very few of these books had been empirically tested and that nearly one fifth contained treatment recommendations that might actually be harmful, such as overstated claims about alternative or untested treatments (Redding et al., in press). Even worse, some books advocated for treatment techniques that have been shown to exacerbate symptoms!

As such, we focus our review on books that have the greatest empirical base. Most studies have focused on one of two books: *Feeling Good* by David Burns, M.D. (1980; 1999a), and *Control Your Depression* by Peter Lewinsohn, Ph.D., Ricardo Muñoz, Ph.D., Mary Ann Youngren, Ph.D., and Antonette Zeiss, Ph.D. (1978; 1992). We will review the evidence for each of these books below along with a section describing studies using other bibliotherapy approaches. Unless noted, all studies are randomized controlled trials deemed to be of high quality in a previous meta-analysis using relatively rigorous standards (den Boer et al., 2004). These book titles are listed in a hand-out for patients listing publicly available self-help resources (see Table 4.1).

Feeling Good

Feeling Good was first published in 1980 but is currently available in a mass-market paperback book that was updated in 1999 (Burns, 1999a). A second book entitled *The Feeling Good Handbook* (Burns, 1999b) is also available, which contains additional techniques for depression as well as techniques for anxiety management and improved communication skills. This version of the book also contains strategies for therapists using the book that will be discussed in a later section of this chapter. We will focus here on the original *Feeling Good*, as it is the book used in the research studies summarized below.

This book presents a self-assessment of depression symptoms and then provides education about the cognitive model of depression. With user-friendly language and activities, later chapters include instructions for clients to apply cognitive behavioral therapy (CBT) techniques, including challenging automatic thoughts ("Start by Building Self-Esteem"), behavioral activation ("Do-Nothingism: How to Beat it"), and cognitive restructuring of core beliefs and schema as a form of relapse prevention ("Prevention and Personal Growth"). The book also includes strategies for coping with criticism and managing anger, guilt, hopelessness, and stress. The 1999 edition concludes with information about antidepressant medication and the biological basis of depression.

Several studies have supported the efficacy of reading *Feeling Good* as an approach to reducing depression symptoms. In these studies, participants are typically given 1 month to read the book and complete the exercises. They receive weekly phone contact with a therapist or researcher who provides brief assessment and answers questions about the book. However, these calls do not contain counseling and are typically 5 to 15 minutes. However, it is also worth noting that *Feeling Good* has also been applied as a 10-week seminar in which participants read *Feeling Good* and completed CBT homework assignments outside of group meetings (Bright et al., 1999). This program has also been found to be effective in producing clinically significant reductions in depression. (We will revisit this study in more detail in Chapter 7, as it speaks to the issue of the efficacy of therapy delivered by paraprofessional therapists. For now, we will

Table 4.1 Self-help resources for patients

Websites that provide reliable information on depression:
BluePages – psychoeducational information about depression
http://www.bluepages.anu.edu.au/

The MacArther Initiative on Depression – patient education on depression
http://www.depression-primarycare.org/clinicians/toolkits/materials/patient_edu/

Here to Help – Toolkit for managing depression, with an interactive version
http://www.heretohelp.bc.ca/skills/managing-depression

National Institute of Mental Health – Resources in English and Spanish
http://www.nimh.nih.gov/health/topics/depression/index.shtml

Medline Plus – Additional resources in English and Spanish
http://www.nlm.nih.gov/medlineplus/depression.html

Depression and Bipolar Support Alliance (DBSA)
http://www.dbsalliance.org/site/PageServer?pagename=about_depression_overview

Websites that provide self-screening for depression:
The Center for Epidemiological Studies Depression Scale (CES-D)
http://med.stanford.edu/patienteducation/research/cesd.pdf
http://www.intelihealth.com/IH/ihtIH/WSIHW000/23722/9025.html

Patient Health Questionnaire
http://www.depression-primarycare.org/clinicians/toolkits/materials/forms/phq9/

Quick Inventory of Depressive Symptomatology Self-Report (QIDS-SR)
http://www.dbsalliance.org/site/PageServer?pagename=about_depressionscreener

Self-help books:
Control Your Depression by Peter Lewinsohn, Ph.D., Ricardo Muñoz, Ph.D., Mary Ann Youngren, Ph.D., and Antonette Zeiss, Ph.D. (1978).

Feeling Good by David Burns, M.D. (1999a).

Mind Over Mood by Dennis Greenberger, Ph.D. and Christine Padesky (1995).

Computerized cognitive-behavioral psychotherapy programs:
Overcoming Depression on the Internet (**ODIN**)
http://www.kpchr.org/feelbetter/

MoodGYM
http://www.moodgym.anu.edu.au/welcome

MySelfHelp.com
http://www.myselfhelp.com/Programs/DD.html

---

focus on studies in which the bibliotherapy is administered with the individual, self-administered paradigm described above.)

In a study of older adults with one or more disability in activity of daily living and diagnosed with a depressive disorder, participants were randomly assigned to a minimal contact condition (reading *Feeling Good* and brief weekly telephone call from researchers without counseling) or a delayed treatment waitlist (Landreville & Bissonnette, 1997). After 4 weeks, the treated group showed modest improvement in depression symptoms. At a 6-month follow-up of all participants (both groups had received treatment at this point), depression symptom reductions were maintained and reductions in "excess disability" (i.e. patient does not perform tasks they are physically capable of doing) were also observed.

In a second study (Scogin et al.,1987) of mild to moderately depressed older adults, bibliotherapy (*Feeling Good* read under conditions similar to the above study) was found to be superior to two control conditions: a delayed-treatment waitlist and attention placebo, in this case reading *Man's Search for Meaning* by Viennese psychiatrist Victor Frankl (1959). This book is an inspiring and widely read book consisting of Frankl's memoir of surviving internment in a Nazi concentration camp and his discussion of how this experience shaped his approach to psychotherapy; however, the book does not contain formal educational material about depression or structured self-help exercises. This study suggests that a CBT self-help book may have benefits above and beyond reading a book presenting a vivid account of adjustment to adversity and discussing psychotherapy in more abstract terms.

In a later study testing the relative efficacy of *Feeling Good*, mildly to moderately depressed older adults were randomly assigned to read *Feeling Good* or *Control Your Depression* during a 1-month period with brief, non-counseling weekly phone contact. Participants in both groups experienced greater reductions in depression symptoms than those on a 1-month waitlist (Scogin et al., 1989). The books did not differ in terms of efficacy, and gains appeared to be maintained at 6-month and 2-year follow-up periods in both conditions (Scogin et al., 1990). Interestingly, at the 2-year follow-up, most of the participants felt their depression had decreased and had not received other treatment. Just over half of the participants reported having re-read at least part of their assigned book during the 2 years since the study began.

The most rigorous test to date was a comparison of *Feeling Good* bibliotherapy (1 month with brief non-counseling phone follow-up) with 12 weeks of therapist-administered individual CBT and a delayed treatment control group (Floyd et al., 2004). Both interventions were found to be superior to the control condition in the short term. Not surprisingly, participants had improved more in 12 weeks of therapist-administered CBT than in 4 weeks of bibliotherapy. However, at a 3-month follow-up, both groups had achieved comparable improvement. Gains in both groups were maintained at a 2-year follow-up; however, individuals in the bibliotherapy condition had experienced more recurrences of depression in the intervening years (Floyd et al., 2006). A number of those in the bibliotherapy condition reported re-reading the book at different times, including three participants who had experienced a recurrence.

This complex pattern of findings will be discussed in a later section of this chapter focused on remaining questions about bibliotherapy and computerized psychotherapy.

Control Your Depression

Control Your Depression was first published in 1978 and is based on social-learning theory, which suggests that loss of pleasant and increase in unpleasant person–environment interactions plays a role in maintaining depression. The book includes a copy of the Beck Depression Inventory as a self-assessment of depression, along with a presentation of the social-learning theory. Later chapters present guides to relaxation and social skills (particularly assertiveness training), pleasant events scheduling, challenging negative thoughts, and self-instruction. Final chapters focus on relapse prevention, including self-monitoring and goal-setting. Compared with *Feeling Good, Control Your Depression* generally places greater emphasis on traditional behavioral interventions consistent with the social-learning theory that informs the intervention (Scogin et al., 1989). Nonetheless, both books have considerable overlap and, as noted previously, when administered as individual bibliotherapy, both appear to be equally efficacious (Scogin et al., 1989; Scogin et al., 1990).

Control Your Depression is more commonly administered in group format as part of the Coping With Depression psychoeducational course developed by Lewinsohn and colleagues (1984). The course typically consists of 12 sessions with two booster sessions, the group leader acts more like an instructor than a therapist, and recruitment is often through the media to increase outreach to populations who may not be otherwise served. The course has been applied to diverse populations and achieves an overall effect comparable to that of other psychotherapies for depression (Cuijpers, 1998). One study examined whether *Control Your Depression* is any less effective when administered as individual bibliotherapy with minimal contact than when read as part of the Coping with Depression course presented in either group or individual format (Brown & Lewinsohn, 1984). In this study, participants were assigned to either a delayed-treatment waitlist or one of three active treatment conditions consisting of 12 sessions over 8 weeks: (1) the Coping with Depression course presented in group format (more or less as described above), (2) the course presented in individual tutoring sessions lasting roughly 50 minutes, or (3) the minimal contact condition consisting of one in-person meeting with a tutor and the remaining sessions conducted in 20-minute contacts over the telephone. In all conditions, participants were instructed to read *Control Your Depression* and complete the assignments described in the book. All three active treatment conditions were superior to the waitlist control group. Importantly, the minimal contact bibliotherapy condition was equally efficacious to the two interventions involving greater clinician contact at both the post-treatment and 1- and 6-month follow-ups. Of particular note was that of the 14 participants in this condition, only 1 met criteria for depression at the 6-month follow-up. This suggests that patients can receive comparable benefit with reduced clinician time or the potential supportive benefits of a group intervention.

Other bibliotherapy approaches

Mind Over Mood

One book that is widely used as a supplement to CBT psychotherapy is *Mind Over Mood* by Dennis Greenberger, Ph.D., and Christine Padesky (1995). In a recent review of 50 best-selling self-help books, *Mind Over Mood* received generally high ratings across a number of categories, including usefulness, grounding in psychological science, and degree of specific guidance (Redding et al., in press). The book primarily serves as a tutorial in the use of a key CBT intervention: the thought-record used to monitor and challenge negative cognitions. The book contains relatively briefer content on behavioral activation and goal-setting and strategies for coping with anxiety, anger, guilt, and shame relative to *Feeling Good*. An additional benefit of this book is that it is also available in Spanish.

This book has not been subjected to randomized controlled trials. However, one study examined the use of this book as an initial intervention for patients with symptoms of anxiety or depression on a 6-week psychotherapy waitlist (Whitfield et al., 2001). Patients were invited to schedule appointments to read *Mind Over Mood* in a self-help room located in a psychiatric day hospital. Just over half of the invited patients took advantage of this program and attended an average of 3.6 sessions. As a whole, participants in this group experienced reduction in depression and anxiety symptoms and negative cognition and found the program to be acceptable and useful. Conclusions are limited by the lack of a control group. However, this presents an interesting model of how self-help can be integrated into routine care.

Unpublished manuals

Other studies have been conducted using manuals developed for the purpose of the study but that are not published. For instance, a study by Schmidt found that minimal-contact CBT bibliotherapy using a manual developed for the study was equally effective at reducing symptoms of depression as individual or group CBT psychotherapy but superior to a waitlist control group (Schmidt & Miller, 1983). An additional study of patients with depression found that bibliotherapy with minimal contact using an unpublished CBT-based manual developed by the author was superior to a waitlist control group but comparable to two group-based interventions: therapist-delivered CBT and supportive therapies (Wollersheim & Wilson, 1991).

Research on computerized psychotherapy as a treatment for depression

History and background

Computerized psychotherapy was not developed exclusively with the goal of treating and managing depression. As summarized by Cavanagh and Shapiro (2004), the history of computerized psychotherapy roughly mirrors the history of prevailing schools of psychotherapy during the second half of the twentieth century. Beginning in the 1960s, the earliest computer psychotherapy programs used text-generating software to prompt a user to input a statement about what was troubling them, select key phrases of typed input, retrieve a response from a list, and insert fragments from the input into the response. The goal of such programs was to simulate an empathic dialogue typical of humanistic psychotherapy; however, such programs remain more of a novelty than a serious clinical tool. Beginning in the 1970s and 1980s, a second wave of programs inspired by the behavioral movement was designed to guide patients through systematic desensitization for phobias and other anxiety disorders. Although beyond the scope of this chapter on depression treatments, it should be noted that computerized self-help programs for anxiety disorders continue to be developed and have gained considerable research support (see Cavanagh & Shapiro, 2004; Spek et al., 2006; and Walker et al., 2009 for recent reviews).

Beginning in the late 1980s and early 1990s, computer programs emerged that integrated cognitive therapy techniques such as psychoeducation, problem-solving training, and cognitive restructuring. It was during this wave that the first programs to treat depression emerged. These programs were in part inspired by promising results of bibliotherapy for depression.

Early programs were often text-heavy and utilized computer programs stored on a single computer to deliver CBT. Initial studies typically had small samples, and the software did not become widely available beyond the research trial. The current wave of programs for depression typically makes greater use of engaging multi-media presentation formats, including animation, video clips, graphics, and voice-overs as well as interactive exercises. The latest generation of programs have been tested on much larger samples in a variety of settings and are typically available for practitioners and patients on CD-ROM for delivery from a single computer in a clinical setting or on websites that can be accessed 24 hours a day. In Table 4.1, we present a list of Internet-based programs that are available directly to patients. In Table 4.2, we present a more comprehensive

Table 4.2 Summary for clinicians of computerized CBT programs

Program name	RCT?[1]	Format	Is there a cost associated with use?	How to obtain additional information
Beating the Blues	Yes	CD-ROM	Yes	http://www.ultrasis.com/products
Good Days Ahead	Yes	CD-ROM	Yes	http://www.mindstreet.com/
Overcoming Depression on the Internet	Yes	Website	No	http://www.kpchr.org/feelbetter/
MoodGYM	Yes	Website	No	http://www.moodgym.anu.edu.au/welcome
MySelfHelp.com	No	Website	Yes	http://www.myselfhelp.com/Programs/DD.html
Overcoming Depression	No	CD-ROM	Yes	http://www.calipso.co.uk/mainframe.htm
COPE	No	Telephone: Interactive voice response (IVR)	Yes	http://www.healthtechsys.com/products/edcare_cope.html
LifeCoach	No	Website with live help from clinicians available	Yes	http://www2.lifeoptions.com/lifecoach.jsp

[1] RCT? = Has the program been supported by the results of at least one randomized controlled trial (RCT)?

list of currently available programs that can be purchased and administered by clinicians and organizations.

Summary of research

This section will review the empirical support for computerized psychotherapy programs for depression. As noted previously, nearly all are based on a CBT model, which is didactic and skills-based and therefore lends itself to computerized psychotherapy. This review will focus on programs that have been tested with randomized controlled trials because this type of study provides the strongest evidence that computerized psychotherapy directly leads to symptom improvement. However, several uncontrolled studies have been conducted that offer useful information about the "real-world" effectiveness of these programs. Some of these studies will be discussed in the later section on practical recommendations.

This section will first discuss non-Internet–based computerized therapies – programs delivered on a single computer terminal, often located in a clinical setting. We will then review programs delivered over the Internet to provide CBT and psychoeducation about depression.

Non-Internet–based computerized psychotherapies

The first major studies of computerized cognitive behavioral therapy (CBT) appeared in the prestigious *American Journal of Psychiatry* in 1990 (Selmi et al., 1990). The study compared the efficacy of 6 sessions of computerized CBT, therapist-delivered CBT, and a waitlist control group in a sample of 36 outpatients with depressive disorders. The computer program provided an orientation to CBT, administered and scored the Beck Depression Inventory each week, provided feedback on symptom severity and week-to-week change, asked patients to generate a problem list, and provided interactive activities to demonstrate CBT techniques such as challenging automatic thoughts. The program also gave homework assignments, including additional reading and CBT activities tailored to the content of the session (e.g. monitoring automatic thoughts, scheduling activities likely to produce feelings of mastery and pleasure). An experimenter was available to answer questions about the computer program. In the therapy condition, patients received six sessions of CBT following a protocol similar to the computer program. Both the computer program and therapist-delivered CBT were effective at reducing depression symptoms, yet neither demonstrated superior efficacy. Two later studies of inpatients with depression using the program described above (Selmi et al., 1990) and a second program (Colby, 1995) tended to show some improvement in symptoms, but these were comparable to changes in control groups receiving treatment as usual (Bowers et al., 1993) or a "placebo" computer therapy (Stutzke et al., 1997).

Taken together, these earlier studies show that patients assigned to computerized therapy do tend to show improvement, but provide mixed evidence of efficacy beyond control conditions particularly for inpatients. Neither of these programs (Colby, 1995; Selmi et al., 1990) were used again in published research, nor are they currently publicly available. Subsequent to these early programs, two programs, *Beating the Blues* and *Good Days Ahead: The Multimedia Program for Cognitive Therapy*, have been developed that improve upon these earlier, text-heavy programs by making use of new multi-media technology. Unlike prototype programs used in earlier studies, both programs are currently available for use in clinical settings (see Table 4.2).

Beating the Blues (BtB) is an interactive computer program that includes video vignettes presented in eight 50-minute sections that build upon each other. Patients first viewed a 15-minute introductory video. Subsequent sessions presented a range of cognitive (e.g. automatic thoughts, core beliefs, attributional style) and behavioral (e.g. activity scheduling, problem-solving) interventions. Homework assignments are given to be completed between sessions, and progress reports are given to the patient and the general practitioner. The first randomized trial (Proudfoot et al., 2003; Proudfoot et al., 2004) enrolled 274 patients with depression and/or anxiety recruited from general practice (i.e. primary care settings). Patients were assigned to either complete BtB or treatment as usual, including pharmacotherapy or psychotherapy. Computer therapy participants were allowed to take medication during the trial if recommended by their general practitioner. BtB sessions were held at the clinic and a nurse was available to provide brief (maximum of 10 minutes per session) contact per visit, largely to provide technical support. Patients receiving BtB showed greater improvement in depression and anxiety symptoms relative to the treatment-as-usual conditions. Given that many patients in both conditions received pharmacotherapy, this study suggests an additive effect of computerized CBT above and beyond medication alone.

Importantly, BtB treatment was found to be equally effective in reducing symptoms regardless of initial severity or duration of symptoms. Also worth noting is that the majority of the sample included patients in the moderate to severe range. Gains were maintained at a 6-month follow-up. Cost-effectiveness analyses from this trial (McCrone et al., 2004) suggest that BtB is comparable in cost to treatment as usual; however, it has the added bonus of increasing workplace productivity as measured by doctor-certified lost days of work. More recently, a study to test the effectiveness of the treatment in routine care (Cavanagh et al., 2006) found that effect sizes from the randomized trial (Proudfoot et al., 2004) were comparable to results obtained in routine care. This suggests that BtB may be effective in more naturalistic clinical settings as well as under the relatively artificial conditions of a controlled research trial. Based on the accumulated evidence, the National Institute for Health and Clinical Excellence (2006) recently endorsed BtB as a first-line treatment for mild to moderate depression in the UK as a measure to counter the large shortages of trained CBT therapists.

A second program that has been supported in a randomized clinical trial is *Good Days Ahead: The Multimedia Program for Cognitive Therapy.* The program contains interactive self-help exercises to teach cognitive therapy techniques (cognitive restructuring of automatic thoughts, behavioral activation, identifying and modifying core beliefs). The program makes extensive use of video, audio, graphics, and checklists. In this study (Wright et al., 2005), the goal was to use the computer program to reduce rather than eliminate therapist contact with a patient. Outpatients with mild to moderate major depressive disorder (MDD) were randomized to either 9 sessions of standard cognitive therapy (50 minutes with a therapist), 9 sessions of computer-assisted cognitive therapy (25 minutes with therapist, 25 minutes working on computer), or a waitlist condition. Both traditional and computer-assisted cognitive therapies were equally efficacious in reducing depression symptoms, and gains were maintained at a 6-month follow-up. The commercially available version of the program was developed in conjunction with Aaron T. Beck, M.D., the founder of cognitive therapy for depression.

Internet-based therapies

Internet-based interventions offer many of the same advantages of computer-based interventions with the added advantage of increasing access and flexibility in terms of times and locations the programs can be administered. This area of investigation got off to a rocky start, with its first two published studies failing to find an effect for the program. Later studies have included some methodological improvements and found more promising results.

The first such study (Clarke et al., 2002) tested a program called *Overcoming Depression on the Internet (ODIN)*. A large sample of primary care patients with and without a recorded diagnosis of depression were recruited from a Kaiser-Permanente health maintenance organization (HMO) database and randomized to have access to ODIN or a control condition in which they did not have access to ODIN. All participants were allowed to continue with their preexisting treatments for depression. The website was split into seven brief chapters, with topics including self-assessment of mood, identification of unrealistic thoughts, and generation of realistic counter-thoughts. This program contained no behavioral interventions. The chapters included interactive activities with some graphics and non-animated cartoons. The researchers enrolled 299 patients. However, no significant difference was found between the treatment and control groups. The authors attributed this lack of effect to two factors. First, most participants were experiencing relatively severe levels of symptoms at intake. Such a low-intensity intervention was likely insufficient for this sample. Exploratory analyses suggest that those with less severe symptoms may gain some benefit. Second, site usage was overall very low; on average, most only visited the site two to three times. In a follow-up trial (Clarke et al., 2005), the authors used similar methods except they added telephone and postcard reminders to the intervention, which produced the desired effect of increasing site usage. In this trial of 255 patients, the intervention produced a modest effect over the treatment-as-usual condition in terms of reducing depression. In contrast to the first trial, the program was found to be more effective for those with greater symptom severity in this trial. It is worth noting that the majority of participants assigned to ODIN had received standard treatment for depression within the past year; thus the effects of ODIN suggest that Internet-based therapy can be helpful in addition to the effect of standard care.

A null effect was also found in a study of an automated program (Patten, 2003) to prevent depression. The intervention was accessible through the Internet or by phone. It included four content modules: cognitive restructuring techniques, activity levels, sleep hygiene and stimulus control, and alcohol consumption. A total of 786 participants were randomized to receive this program or an information-only control group. However, rates of depression during a 3-month follow-up were comparable in the intervention and control group. No follow-up studies of this program have been published.

A more promising intervention is the extensively researched Australian program *MoodGYM*, which typically consists of five CBT modules including cognitive restructuring, problem-solving training, and pleasant events scheduling along with relaxation and assertiveness training. The first randomized controlled trial of this intervention (Christensen et al., 2004) compared *MoodGYM* and *BluePages*, a psychoeducation-only website with information about the symptoms and treatment of depression, and an attentional control condition. The sample consisted of 525 community participants with elevated depression symptoms. Interestingly, both programs (*MoodGYM* and *BluePages*) were found to significantly reduce depression symptoms relative to the control group, suggesting psychoeducation alone can be helpful in reducing symptoms. However, *MoodGYM* was uniquely helpful for reducing dysfunctional thinking, whereas *BluePages* uniquely increased depression literacy and reduced stigma. In a recent review article (Griffiths & Christensen, 2007), the authors note that the results from this trial appear to have been maintained over a 12-month period. Also, more recent trials have shown promise for *MoodGYM* with adolescents and college students, as well as some evidence for the cost-effectiveness of the program.

The website has been publicly available for several years. The benefits obtained by spontaneous users appears to be comparable to those seen for participants enrolled in trials (who received weekly reminders to visit the site). However, the compliance rate was considerably lower among spontaneous users (Christensen et al., 2004). This is important in light of findings that longer exposure to the program is associated with greater improvement in symptoms (Christensen et al., 2002; Christensen et al., 2004). Given that users of the *MoodGYM* website are free to navigate through the pages and select which modules they wish to use, it is important to determine whether smaller doses of the program are as effective as the full program. One study randomized a large sample (N = 2794) of willing visitors to the website to one of six versions of the program of differing length and combinations of modules (Christensen et al., 2006). The two versions of the program that included an extended explanation of cognitive behavioral therapy (CBT) were more effective than those consisting of brief introductions to CBT. However, a version of the program containing all modules (including extended CBT) performed relatively poorly. Results suggest there may be an optimal dose of online CBT; however, conclusions are difficult to draw given that all conditions suffered considerable attrition – as much as 95% in several conditions.

Another online program has shown promising results by integrating minimal contact with a therapist via email. A Swedish study (Andersson et al., 2005) randomized 117 individuals with mild to moderate depression to complete this program and a web-based discussion group or a web-based discussion group only. The program consisted of 89 pages of text that could be printed off for later review, with modules focusing on behavioral activation, cognitive restructuring, sleep and physical health, relapse prevention, and setting future goals. There was a quiz at the end of each module. The results of the quiz were sent to a study therapist who sent feedback within 24 hours and gave the patient access to the next module. The participants also took part in a closely monitored online discussion with other participants. The authors estimate that the therapist spent roughly 2 hours per patient enrolled in this roughly 10-week trial completing screenings, responding to emails, and monitoring discussion groups. At the end of the trial, the treatment group had shown significantly more improvement in depression symptoms than the group who only participated in the discussion group. The control group was allowed to complete the intervention after the initial trial, and at follow-up, both groups demonstrated improvement relative to their initial symptom scores.

In addition to the programs reviewed above, there are many promising web-based CBT for depression programs that have been developed by private entities. These programs often feature similar features of existing programs as well as cutting-edge features to increase their utility and attractiveness to consumers and health care professionals. We will summarize some of these innovations in a later section on the use of self-help resources as part of integrated e-health systems for self-management and communication with clinicians. However, we will not extensively review all available programs for two reasons. First, these programs often do not have the same evidence base in terms of con-trolled trials published in peer-reviewed journals. Second, many programs are not available directly to consumers but instead are marketed to other businesses who, in turn, provide them to employees or subscribers of a health plan. Instead, we will review one of the more well-developed web-based programs, which is directly available to consumers as well as businesses: MySelfHelp.com (www.MySelfHelp.com).

MySelfHelp.com includes modules for depression as well as frequently comorbid disorders and clinical problems including anxiety/stress, grief, insomnia, eating disorders, compulsive shopping, guilt, self-esteem, and HIV. Caregiver support programs and tools are also included. The program includes interactive programs to help users apply CBT skills. For instance, participants can enter a negative thought (e.g. "the future is hopeless") and then are guided to recognize possible cognitive distortions and review evidence that contradicts the thought. A list of adaptive responses to common negative thoughts is presented. Participants can select those that are most helpful to them, and these favorite responses can be re-accessed when the user returns to the site. A unique feature is a calendar on which users can schedule behavioral homework and then receive emailed reminders to complete these self-assignments.

The program can be used as a stand-alone intervention but can also be easily integrated into standard care. Providers may refer patients to the site, and clients are encouraged to share summary results of their usage (e.g. self-assessments, homework results) with their clinicians. The website includes a tip-sheet for clinicians who wish to integrate the program by matching treatment goals with relevant skills modules from MySelfHelp.com.

Patients can access the site by paying a monthly subscription fee. Information entered by users is stored indefinitely. Thus a user may subscribe for a period of time, discontinue use of the program during periods of recovery, and then re-subscribe should symptoms return and pick up where he/she left off.

In 2006, MySelfHelp.com was acquired by HealthMedia, Inc., a company known for providing web-based behavioral health assessment and intervention programs to health plans, employers, pharmaceutical companies, and behavioral health organizations. As such, MySelfHelp.com is now available to employees of some organizations and customers of managed health care organizations, including Kaiser Permanente and some Blue Cross plans, as well as consumers who subscribe through the website.

The program has been the focus of extensive input by mental health specialists, including leading CBT developers and researchers. However, no formal research evaluations of the program have been published. Rich Bedrosian, Ph.D., the founder of MySelfHelp.com, indicates that several non-controlled studies have been conducted and the results are being prepared for publication. Individuals using the program tend to experience reductions in depression symptoms, increased confidence in their ability to manage depression, and improvements in self-rated workplace productivity (R. Bedrosian, personal communication, March, 2008).

Critiques of studies and remaining questions about bibliotherapy and computerized psychotherapy

Taken together, the results of the reviewed studies suggest that bibliotherapy and computerized psychotherapy can be an effective tool for reducing depression. In general, findings suggest that self-help is preferable when professional help is not available. However, it is most likely to work best when integrated within some clinical contact rather than as a fully stand-alone intervention. This is consistent with a self-management perspective where the clinician and patient form a collaborative partnership. In this section, we will discuss the issue of whether self-help therapies (with or without minimal clinician contact) are indeed equally efficacious as therapist-delivered therapies, as some lines of evidence suggest. We will also discuss some of the limitations in studies on self-help and the questions that they raise.

Are self-help therapies equally efficacious as therapist-delivered therapies? Some lines of evidence suggest yes. As noted previously, the overall effect size of bibliotherapies is generally comparable to the effect size found in meta-analyses of studies of therapist-delivered cognitive behavioral therapy (CBT) for depression (den Boer et al., 2004). We also reviewed several studies suggesting that bibliotherapy with minimal clinician contact was equally effective as therapist-delivered individual and group interventions for depression (Brown & Lewinsohn, 1984; Floyd et al., 2004; Floyd et al., 2006; Schmidt & Miller, 1983; Wollersheim & Wilson, 1991). A caveat noted previously is that one study found that although patients who received psychotherapy reported similar symptom levels at 2-year follow-up to patients who received bibliotherapy, therapist-delivered CBT provided better protection against recurrence during those 2 years. Although the bibliotherapy appeared to be an enduring resource for a number of patients, including those who experience recurrence (Floyd et al., 2004; Floyd et al., 2006), these results suggest some trade-offs in terms of durability of bibliotherapy relative to therapist-delivered CBT. More studies are needed that track long-term recurrence in addition to symptoms at a single time of assessment.

The evidence for the relative equal efficacy of computerized psychotherapy and therapist-administered psychotherapy is much more scant. Some advocates of computerized CBT cite the Selmi et al. (1990) study as evidence that computerized therapy is equally effective as therapist-delivered CBT. However, it is worth noting that a second less-frequently cited study found therapist-delivered CBT to be superior to different computerized CBT programs (Bowers et al., 1993). It is important to remember that both studies included very small sample sizes, and surprisingly, no further direct comparisons of computerized versus therapist-delivered psychotherapy have been conducted. There is also some question about the quality of the psychotherapy delivered in these studies. In the Selmi et al. (1990) study, the therapist was restricted to the same content and an equal number of sessions as the computer program, a total of six sessions. On the one hand, this methodological precision is essential to help the researchers control for the effects of time and content in accounting for improvement in symptoms. However, these studies result in a potentially artificial version of therapist-delivered CBT. Future studies are needed in which therapists are given the flexibility to deliver CBT or other forms of psychotherapy in a manner typical of real clinical settings. Similar critiques may be applied to the abbreviated therapy included in some bibliotherapy studies. Importantly, most patients have been found to show a preference for therapist-delivered interventions over computerized interventions (Marks et al., 2003).

Another issue that raises questions about the feasibility of stand-alone computerized psychotherapy is a consistent pattern of findings that attrition rates tend to increase as the amount of clinician support or study structure decreases. In studies in which outpatients complete computerized therapy in a clinic in the context of research studies, rates of attrition are often quite low, for example, 0% in the Selmi et al. (1990) study to 13% in Wright et al. (2005). In more naturalistic studies, rates of non-completion are as high as 50% (Marks et al., 2003; van den Berg et al., 2004). Internet-based studies have reported attrition rates as low as 21% in a trial that included reminder calls from interviewers (Christensen et al., 2004) and 35% in a trial in which participants received reminder postcards or telephone calls (Clarke et al., 2005). A similar rate of attrition (37%) was found in a study in which participants also received email contact from a therapist (Andersson et al., 2005). In a more recent study that did not include reminder calls, 70% to 80% of participants who completed an initial assessment session failed to return to a second session; only 5% of those assigned to a multi-session intervention completed the intervention (Christensen et al., 2006). This latter finding underscores that, without automated reminders or contact with study staff or clinicians, compliance rates with web-based interventions may be very low. Indeed, bibliotherapy studies tend to have lower attrition rates, and this may be due in part to the use of minimal-clinician contact in the form of brief, weekly telephone appointments.

High attrition rates raise several issues. First, from a methodological perspective, it can have the effect of favorably skewing results. Because assessments in most studies were contingent on participating in treatment, more data are only available for those who adhere to the program. Many of the published studies report analyses that account for this issue in looking at immediate outcomes; however, follow-up data are only available for a small subset of participants, which may present results biased towards more engaged and motivated participants. A more practical concern regarding high attrition rates is that it can be seen as an indication of low patient satisfaction with the programs. One danger of disseminating treatments that have low adherence rates is that for some users, this may be their first experience with mental health treatment. If it is not sufficiently engaging, it may discourage them from attempting more conventional treatments in the future.

However, there are other ways of interpreting this high attrition rate for Internet-based programs. In contrast to typical randomized controlled trials, attrition in web-based interventions is much higher, as patients have received far less clinical filtering and follow-up. Thus it is easy both to enroll and to drop out. Also, many participants may only be seeking information or enroll out of curiosity (Christensen et al., 2006). As such, a website that provides reliable information about depression would not be considered a failure if a patient only visited it once after receiving the information they needed. It is also possible that a subset of drop-outs are those who do improve and, feeling they have gotten all the benefit they can from the program, do not return for later sessions or follow-up assessments.

Other methodological limitations of studies of Internet-based interventions should be noted. Samples are rarely well-characterized, meaning that enrollment is often open to those with elevated depression symptoms on a brief self-report depression score (Andersson, 2006; Spek et al., 2006). For pragmatic reasons, interviews to confirm diagnosis are rarely included due to the large numbers of participants who enroll and the desire to guarantee participants anonymity. Nonetheless, this does limit the degree to which practitioners can feel confident that results of Internet-based psychotherapy will generalize to individuals who meet criteria for major depressive disorder (MDD). In contrast, bibliotherapy studies tend to make use of more rigorous structured diagnostic procedures.

A critique that is often raised against many studies of psychosocial interventions is the issue of the adequacy of blinding of treatment conditions. In medication studies using a placebo condition, it is relatively easy to implement a double-blind study. In contrast, while blinded assessments are becoming more common in studies of psychosocial interventions, participants are rarely blind as to whether they are receiving the experimental treatment. This is due in part to the challenge of developing credible "placebo" psychotherapies. Indeed, den Boer and colleagues (2004) note that most bibliotherapy studies have inadequate concealment of randomization, which can inflate effect sizes. It is worth noting that one study found that patients assigned to receive bibliotherapy using *Feeling Good* (which contained "active" CBT ingredients) received greater benefits than those who received equal clinical attention but who were assigned to read an engaging, psychology-oriented book without these ingredients (*Man's Search For Meaning*). Future studies of bibliotherapy and computerized psychotherapy would benefit from the inclusion of similarly credible but presumably inactive treatments. Indeed, the nearly 2000 self-help books published each year (Rosen, 1993) provide ample possibilities!

In summary, bibliotherapy for depression tends to have a more solid base of evidence and greater methodological rigor than studies of Internet-based therapies. Given that Internet-based therapy is still a relatively new and rapidly evolving area of inquiry, some of the limitations noted above may be addressed in future studies as researchers employ increasingly sophisticated methods. Nonetheless, bibliotherapy and computerized psychotherapy represent a dramatic enough departure from standard methods of delivering care that they raise several pragmatic challenges to implementation. The following section addresses these concerns regarding the cost of computerized psychotherapy and the attitudes of clinicians and patients towards self-help.

Practical challenges to implementing bibliotherapy and computerized psychotherapy

Cost of self-help to clinicians and patients

There are many arguments that bibliotherapy and computerized psychotherapy are cost-effective. Patients receiving self-help psychotherapy may use less of more costly services such as psychopharmacological treatments and therapist-delivered psychotherapy. Successfully treating depression can also reduce the costs of medical treatments for diseases worsened by depression, such as heart disease and diabetes. If self-help programs are found to be effective in preventing relapse, this could translate into savings on the cost of later treatment of acute episodes. Successfully and inexpensively treating depression also can produce societal savings in terms of increased workplace productivity. Research has supported some of these claims of cost-effectiveness of bibliotherapy (Vos et al., 2005) and computerized psychotherapy (Griffiths & Christensen, 2007; McCrone et al., 2004). What is not typically considered is the cost to clinicians and patients of implementing some forms of computerized therapy.

In most clinical studies, computerized psychotherapy is only offered for the duration of the study. The cost of developing, licensing, and staffing the technology is typically covered by research grants and, in some cases, the software being donated by for-profit companies with the incentive of later marketing the software commercially. However, for the clinician interested in implementing computer-based psychotherapy outside of the context of grant-funded research or a private software development firm, there are several costs. First, for most software, there is typically a cost associated with licensing the software itself, and there may be additional programming costs associated with adapting the software to a new setting. Second, if the clinician plans to deliver the treatment at their clinic, there is the cost of purchasing computers and training staff who will oversee use of the program. Third, designating space in a clinic for computer usage may potentially limit the number of rooms that can be used for billable services. One alternative to having the clinician's practice absorb the costs of computerized therapies is asking patients to pay out of pocket for the enhanced convenience of computerized therapy. It is unlikely that insurance companies will reimburse for this cost; therefore, this may limit access to computerized psychotherapy for those who can afford additional treatment expenses. However, insurance providers and HMOs are increasingly providing access to computerized self-help programs to its members for no additional charge. In addition, the costs associated with physically housing computerized self-help programs in clinics may be increasingly less relevant given the increased access to computers and the Internet in homes, workplaces, and other public facilities.

Concerns about costs to patients need not prevent clinicians from recommending self-help. Clinicians can refer patients to free web-based interventions listed in Tables 4.1 and 4.2 to supplement standard treatment. Patients willing to pay may seek out commercially available websites offering to treat depression (e.g. MySelfHelp.com, which offers many features not available in free programs). Alternatively, bibliotherapy typically translates into negligible added cost, as the two most widely studied books (*Feeling Good* and *Control Your Depression*) are available in inexpensive paperback editions.

It is also important to realize that patients and clinicians are not the only stakeholders in the cost of treatments for depression. Insurance companies, HMOs, and employers are also motivated to keep down costs of mental health care. Indeed, many insurance companies provide patients with information about depression on their websites. In fact, as noted previously, some HMOs have integrated Internet-based computerized psychotherapy into the services offered to its customers. As such, systemic changes in the ways individuals access mental health care may shape the use of self-help more than the behavior of individual clinicians.

Potential resistance from psychotherapists

From an ethical perspective, the first-line treatments for patients should have minimal cost and burden with maximum availability and efficacy. Self-help programs have the promise of providing patients with an inexpensive, non-invasive, and easily accessible treatment for which there is increasing evidence of its efficacy. Therefore, an argument can be made that such approaches are in a patient's best interest. Why would any clinician neglect a patient's best interest?

John Norcross, Ph.D., a former president of the American Psychological Association and noted self-help researcher, notes that "many mental health professionals maintain an ambivalent, hostile-dependent relationship with self-help. We recommend it, but still mistrust it" (Norcross, 2006; p 684). He notes the roots of this may be a desire to view their services as valuable and fears of economic survival. Some psychotherapists may fear that computerized programs will make their jobs obsolete. One argument against this doomsday scenario comes from Dr. Warner Slack (2001), a physician, Harvard Medical School professor, and pioneer in the integration of computers into health care who said that "any doctor who can be replaced by a computer should be." This quote suggests that skilled clinicians can do things computers cannot do and therefore will always be needed. In Chapter 1, we discussed that clinical care and self-management complement rather than replace one another. In Chapter 2, we described some of the unique and necessary roles that clinicians play which cannot be replaced with self-management tools, including making challenging differential diagnoses, providing empathic understanding, troubleshooting, and adjusting a treatment plan when initial treatments are not successful. As such, we believe the future of computerized interventions is likely to enhance clinician-delivered treatment, not replace it.

Nonetheless, there remains a pragmatic incentive barrier for some clinicians. One public policy argument for self-help is that there are shortages of trained mental health professionals; therefore, adoption of computerized psychotherapy can increase the number of patients any one clinician can serve (Marks et al., 2003). From a clinician's perspective, an expanded caseload can feel more like a liability than an incentive. With larger caseloads, clinicians may not get to know their patients as well. As a result, care could become less personalized and patients at risk for suicide or other dangerous behavior may more easily slip through the cracks. Further, the costs in terms of time and resources devoted to adopting new technologies and the potential lost revenue of reducing the number of patient contacts may present clear disincentives for clinicians in private practices. However, these concerns must also be balanced by what is best for the patients. We have described many of the potential benefits to patients of integrating self-help into clinical care. It is also important to recognize that professions evolve, adapt, and can even benefit from new technologies and changes in the market forces. As such, for clinicians who find themselves stuck viewing self-help as a "threat," we recommend the following two minor cognitive-restructuring interventions for reframing it as an "opportunity."

As managed health care session limits and patients' busy life schedules force clinicians to fit effective treatment into increasingly fewer face-to-face minutes, self-help interventions may allow clinicians to delegate routine aspects of care and help clinicians deliver the aspects of care they are uniquely qualified to provide. Similarly, if patients complete computerized psychotherapy units before sessions, they may be better prepared to engage with psychotherapy when they arrive for the session. Like a college seminar, the most substantive and rewarding discussions occur when students have done the assigned reading in advance. In summary, computerized psychotherapy could actually make the limited face-to-face session time more rewarding for clinician and patient.

As for concerns about lost revenue, a contrasting perspective is that adding computerized psychotherapy may make a practice more marketable. As we have noted previously, self-help is intrinsically appealing to many individuals (Norcross, 2006). A psychotherapy practice which offers the autonomy, convenience, and cost savings of self-help coupled with the expertise and safety that comes with professional care may attract individuals who might not otherwise be open to seeking professional help. This is consistent with the model of the psychoeducational Coping with Depression courses described earlier. Indeed, self-help programs featuring self-scoring assessment tools will increase awareness of symptoms in the general public and increase the number of individuals who seek services. This is consistent with our experiences in a study we have described earlier in which introducing depression screening in primary care settings led to an increase in referrals for treatment.

For clinicians who are now ready to embrace self-help in their practice, in the following sections, we offer suggestions on how to do so.

Practical recommendations for incorporating bibliotherapy and computerized psychotherapy into a treatment plan

As we have reviewed in the preceding sections, bibliotherapy and computerized psychotherapy shows promise as a treatment for depression and as a potential form of self-management, especially when combined with some clinician contact. In the following section, we discuss practical recommendations for integrating self-help into a treatment plan. This section is divided into two sections. The first section reviews initial decisions providers should make about to whom they may wish to recommend self-help and how to be effective in supporting use of self-help. The second section describes four possible scenarios for integrating self-help into various stages of depression treatment based upon published accounts.

Initial decisions

To whom should self-help be recommended?

Given that this is a relatively new area of research, there are not yet any consistent findings about what kind of patients tend to do best in self-help. One meta-analysis found a relatively larger effect size for bibliotherapy treatments in adolescents and younger adults compared with elderly individuals, suggesting that bibliotherapy may be more effective in younger participants (Gregory et al., 2004). However, the authors caution that this result may be an artifact of the small number of studies examined and the relatively lower levels of symptom severity in the elderly sample at the beginning of treatment, and thus less able to show the effects of the treatment. A study of mildly depressed college students who completed a CBT bibliotherapy for depression found that individuals with higher self-efficacy and a more "realistic" personality type (introverted, mechanically inclined, and practical) showed the greatest improvements in symptoms (Mahalik & Kivlighan, 1998). Such individuals were also more likely to be satisfied with the self-help treatment and prefer self-help to therapist-administered treatments. Although there are questions about whether these findings can be applied to individuals with clinically significant depression, they suggest that some individuals may be better suited to this type of approach.

Bearing in mind that volunteers for studies of computerized psychotherapy are a self-selected group, they are likely comfortable using computers and are somewhat self-motivated. Therefore, such programs may not be appropriate for those who struggle with computers or are less motivated. The effort required to complete a computerized therapy program was found to be a primary reason of drop-out in one study that systematically tracked factors contributing to attrition (Andersson et al., 2005). As all programs involve varying degree of text, basic reading ability is required. Also, CBT in any format requires some self-awareness and ability to apply abstract concepts. Therefore, the psychological mindedness of the patient should be considered.

Most studies of bibliotherapy have been with patients experiencing mild to moderate depression symptoms, and this may be the most appropriate group given the relatively lower risk of suicidal behavior or severe impairment in motivation and attention (Gregory et al., 2004). It is worth noting that bibliotherapy for depression and anxiety do not appear to be less effective in samples with more severe symptoms, as indexed by chronicity of symptoms or history of previous treatment (den Boer et al., 2004). No discernible pattern in the literature suggests whether computerized psychotherapy should be recommended for patients with more severe depression. Studies have found each possible result: patients with mild depression do better (Clarke et al., 2002), patients with more severe depression do better (Clarke et al., 2005), and initial severity is not predictive of outcomes (Proudfoot et al., 2004). At present, clinical judgment is likely to be more useful than cut-off scores in making this determination. In reviewing the literature on self-help in general for depression, Mains and Scogin (2003) caution that self-help tends to be less effective for depressed patients with personality disorders or interpersonal problems. Indeed, most bibliotherapy studies screen-out individuals with comorbid conditions (Gregory et al., 2004). For instance, one clinic-based program testing the "real-world" effectiveness of computerized CBT for depression and anxiety screened patients for suitability factors, including suicide risk, motivation, and applicability of CBT for the patient's presenting problem (Marks et al., 2003).

As noted previously, bibliotherapy and computerized therapy may be especially promising in overcoming some of the barriers to treatment. As such, these approaches may be particularly appropriate for individuals who live in geographically remote areas. Similarly, they may be especially helpful for individuals unwilling to take medication or receive psychotherapy due to cultural stigma associated with receiving mental health services.

Interventions relying on self-help with minimal clinician contact may not be consistent with patient's conceptualization of psychotherapy. Qualitative results suggest some patients seek out therapy to gain "insight" into their problems, whereas self-help programs tend to focus primarily on symptom resolution (MacDonald et al., 2007). In some cases, clinicians may be able to help address this expectancy gap initially. However, some patients may still prefer an insight-oriented therapy. Alternately, some patients may not take readily to the overtly educational nature of self-help programs such as computerized CBT and may gain more from other forms of self-help, such as attending self-help groups or reading autobiographies of individuals who successfully coped with depression (Norcross, 2006), an intriguing suggestion awaiting empirical study. As such, before recommending a self-help program, clinicians should first assess patient's own expectancies and preferences for the format of psychotherapy. If a patient does not accept the idea of bibliotherapy or computerized psychotherapy, it is unlikely to be effective.

Decide on the clinician's role

In the following section, we discuss four models for using self-help interventions. Each includes varying roles for clinicians. Therefore, it is important for the therapist to have a clear conceptualization of the role of the book or computer program in the treatment plan and their role in supporting it. Regardless of role, there are likely several responsibilities that will befall the clinician recommending or supervising a patient's use of self-help. As Gregory and colleagues (2004) note, the clinician plays a crucial role in whether the patient is a good match for self-help interventions, determining how the self-help materials are to be used, including which book or computer program is likely to be best and which assignments would be most relevant. During meetings with the patient, the clinician can clarify concepts and skills and help the patient apply them to his/her own situation and provide motivation and encouragement.

If self-help assignments are being recommended prior to contact with a psychotherapist (for instance, for patients on a psychotherapy waitlist), it is important that the patients know that their concerns are in fact being taken seriously (Scogin et al., 2003). It is important to clearly explain the reason the computer program is being recommended; for instance, to provide an immediate resource while waiting for a live psychotherapist or for medication to take effect. As a practical matter, the clinician should be prepared to address privacy concerns about who will have access to the information patients enter into computerized programs.

As with any treatment, it is important that a clinician be able to express confidence that the program will be helpful for the patient. This may include mentioning research studies supporting the assigned book or program. Also, clinicians need to have some self-awareness of any of their own negative attitudes towards self-help which may be evident in communications with patients. Norcross (2006) notes that many clinicians – psychotherapists in particular – may be inclined to devalue or mistrust self-help programs. If this skepticism is based on limits in the research to date, it may be helpful to present patients with this balanced picture. However, if these attitudes are based in "professional-centrism" (i.e. only trained psychotherapists can help facilitate change), it may be important to remember that clinicians have a skewed base of experiences. Self-help programs are widely used; however, people who recover entirely on their own are invisible to clinicians, as they do not typically present for treatment (Norcross, 2006).

As with all self-management prescriptions, it is valuable to ask patients about their history with book or computer self-help. For instance, many patients will seek information about depression on the web and may have had a negative experience or received inaccurate, anecdotal information from a website or Internet-based chat room. They may have read non-scientifically based self-help books in which authors set unrealistic expectations for success and fail to prepare the patient for the potential of relapse (Redding et al., in press). Therefore, clinicians may need to take time to distinguish the book or computer program they are recommending from non-scientifically based resources and possibly re-moralize patients to give bibliotherapy or computerized self-help another try.

As we have noted several times, self-help programs appear to be most effective with some degree of human support for most patients. Therefore, the clinician who recommends self-help should be prepared to provide some support and enhance motivation for engaging with the program. With each patient contact, it is important to ask at least briefly about the patient's use of the assigned program, address any concerns, and troubleshoot around barriers in using the program. A clinician should also have some familiarity with the program and be prepared to answer questions about its content. Some books and computer programs have supplemental resources for clinicians. However, it is likely valuable for the clinician to actually try out the program to gain first-hand knowledge. If face-to-face visits will be infrequent, consider working with the patient to develop an acceptable reminder system for using the program, such as a phone call from an office staff member or an automated email message.

Models for integrating self-help in practice

In this section, we discuss four possible models for integrating self-help into practice. In the first model, self-help is offered to a patient before or instead of psychotherapy or, in some cases, medication. In the second model, self-help is presented as a "therapist extender," in which self-help is presented along with abbreviated psychotherapy. In the third model, self-help is presented as a complement to standard psychotherapy. In the final approach, self-help is integrated into a comprehensive e-health system that also provides assessment and information and facilitates communication between patients and clinicians. Although presented separately, these models are not mutually exclusive, and interested clinicians may pick and choose components of each that they feel may be most useful for their practice. Similarly, most of these strategies are not specific to any one book or computerized psychotherapy program.

Self-help as a first step in a stepped-care model

One model is to provide self-help as a first step in a stepped-care model. Stepped-care is characterized by providing the least intensive treatment as a first-line approach, progress is monitored, and patients needing additional treatment are "stepped up" to a more intensive treatment (Bower & Gilbody, 2005; Scogin et al., 2003). In this application, patients would be offered bibliotherapy or computerized self-help before being offered face-to-face psychotherapy. This may be attractive to patients in settings when there is limited access to psychotherapy (e.g. a long wait for appointments, insufficient number of providers, geographic and/or language barriers). Similarly, a clinic may elect to use some form of self-help such as bibliotherapy or computerized psychotherapy as a first step with patients with more mild to moderate symptoms and reserve limited clinician-delivered therapies for patients who present with more severe symptoms (Scogin et al., 2003). A physician may refer patients with mild to moderate depression to self-help before prescribing medication if medical factors rule out antidepressant medication as a first-line approach. Another reason to offer self-help interventions would be patient's preference. Such a collaborative approach to care is consistent with the philosophy of self-management.

In this model, the patient might be given access to a computer program in a clinical location or be referred to an Internet-based program. Interestingly, as many as 18.6% of *MoodGYM* users are referred to this program by a health practitioner (Griffiths & Christensen, 2007).

Such a model is illustrated by a report from a community mental health clinic in Doncaster, UK, in which computerized psychotherapy (in this case, the *Beating the Blues* program) was used as treatment for depression and anxiety (van den Berg et al., 2004). When the program was instituted, it had a waitlist of nearly 18 months for a client to be seen by a CBT therapist. Thus use of the program was offered to new patients referred for treatment and those already on the waitlist. At each session, patients were greeted by a "clinical helper" (in this setting, a receptionist) who had received approximately 2 hours of instruction in the use of the program. The clinical helper would orient the patient to the use of the program during the initial meeting (10–15 minutes) and provide a few minutes of support at subsequent sessions, typically involving reminders about use of the computer. In previous clinical trials of this program, a nurse served as the "clinical helper" (e.g. Proudfoot et al., 2004). The authors also recommend that a dedicated room be provided so patients can work without interruption. At each session, the program provides brief assessments of depression, anxiety, and suicidal ideation and sends a report to the referring clinician or the clinician who has responsibility for the patient at the clinic. The authors reported outcomes from a small number of patients suggesting the treatment produced reductions in depression and anxiety symptoms. Forty-five percent of those who began the program did not finish it, but in some cases, this reflects patients who felt they had gained sufficient benefit from a few sessions, according to the authors.

A similar approach was used in testing a new CD-ROM based-program program at a clinic in Glasgow, Scotland (Whitfield et al., 2005). Patients presenting to see a CBT therapist (median wait time was 4 months) were offered the opportunity to use a computerized CBT program called *Overcoming Depression* while they were on the waitlist. Interested patients were instructed to make appointments to use the program at one of three locations (two on a university campus and one in a community health center located in shopping center). A nurse was available during all sessions to provide support in using the program. Patients were informed that their decision would not impact their ability to see a live therapist; however, only one quarter of those asked attended a single session. Of those, 70% completed the program. The program was found to be helpful in producing statistical and clinically significant reductions in depression symptoms. The authors conclude that the uptake rate might be expected to be higher in primary rather than secondary care, in settings with longer waitlists, or when no other form of psychological treatment is available. Although the studies can not be directly compared, Whitfield and colleagues (2001) found higher uptake rates (52%) when giving clients an opportunity to schedule self-administered sessions reading *Mind Over Mood* and completing exercises from the book. As noted in a previous section, the majority of users experienced reductions in symptoms and found the program useful.

These studies offer evidence that integrating self-help as a first-line approach is feasible. In both situations, it is important that some type of support staff is available; however, this service could be provided by a nurse or paraprofessional. Clearly, not all patients will elect to make use of this service. Nonetheless, there is evidence that those who do use these programs appear to experience improvement. As such, it may help to get patients more rapid symptom relief while awaiting other treatment. From these studies, it is unclear whether such a service would lead to patients actually needing fewer sessions of psychotherapy; however, it is a distinct possibility that needs to be examined in future research.

One drawback of the approach taken in these studies is the clinic space needed to be devoted to using the program. On the one hand, having to come to a scheduled appointment to use the programs may provide helpful structure for patients and increase adherence. However, if clinic space is a restraint, patients could be referred to use programs from home. In such situations, it may still be helpful to encourage patients to use them at a scheduled time when a clinic staff member would be available to provide support and answer questions.

Self-help as a therapist extender

In the previous section, we described a model in which patients were given access to self-help before being assigned to a psychotherapist. An alternate model is to assign patients concurrently to computerized treatment and therapist-delivered psychotherapy. In this model, patients meet with therapists for abbreviated sessions, ideally allowing the clinician to serve more clients. Some bibliotherapy programs described earlier make use of psychoeducational groups in which patients are assigned readings between sessions and then meet with a therapist-facilitator to discuss the readings (Bright et al., 1999; Brown & Lewinsohn, 1984). Such an approach extends the therapist by reducing the amount of direct contact with each patient and encourages outside-session learning on the part of the patient.

An intriguing project tested the utility of a free computerized CBT clinic in London to treat depression or anxiety (Gega et al., 2004; Marks et al., 2003). It publicized its services in many places, including primary care offices, psychiatric outpatient clinics, newspaper ads, the yellow pages, and patient organizations. In the 15 months the program was open, the clinic received 355 referrals, screened 266 patients, and enrolled 210 patients deemed appropriate for the services. All referrals were handled by the equivalent of a single full-time nurse and an administrative assistant. Patients were given unlimited access to one of four computerized programs (based on presenting problem) delivered via the Internet, CD-ROM, or telephone-based interactive voice recognition system.

In this study, the primary program for depression patients was the *COPE* program (Osgood-Hynes et al., 1998), a program that provided patients with treatment booklets and telephone calls to a computer-aided interactive voice response (IVR) system. The program consisted of three core modules ("Constructive Thinking," "Pleasant Activities Scheduling," and "Assertive Communication") and provided customized recommendations based on the patient's responses to the IVR questions. Patients read the booklets and then complete interactive activities during the automated phone call. One previous open trial found that patients using *COPE* experienced improvement in their symptoms of depression; however, the program has yet to be tested in a randomized controlled trial.

Patients were scheduled for six brief contacts with a therapist at the clinic in person or over the telephone. Patients could also call the clinician for assistance at other times during business hours. Clinicians did not have access to the content of patients' computerized sessions without patient permission. Aside from the 30-minute screening interview, clinicians had an average of 1 hour of contact with each patient.

The study found clinical and statistically significant improvements for patients using *COPE* and two of the anxiety treatment programs. Roughly 50% of participants completed the recommended course of computerized CBT and provided post-treatment data. The authors report that an additional 30% completed some degree of the programs but did not provide post-treatment data; however, the authors note that some of these individuals had indicated that they felt they had derived benefit from the programs. Patients were generally satisfied with computerized programs, although they had a marginal preference for live therapist support. Unfortunately, after the initial funding for this research project expired, the clinic was not able to obtain additional funding to remain in operation. This reflects the fact that some applications of self-help are radical enough departures from current health care practice that it is likely that health care policy makers will need to be persuaded of the benefits before they can become economically viable. Indeed, it is unclear how clinicians adopting such a model in the United States would be reimbursed.

The experience of this clinic illustrates several pragmatic issues. First, self-help can be used as a clinician extender, consistent with the study of *Good Days Ahead* reviewed earlier (Wright et al., 2005), in which patients met face-to-face with a clinician for 25 minutes and then worked independently on a computer for approximately 25 minutes. In this model, certain aspects of therapy can effectively be delegated to a computer program, and the clinician is reserved for other specialized tasks such as screening interviews and brief counseling. As such, this study suggests a relatively large volume of patients that could be served by a single clinician. This program also suggests that it may also be valuable to also offer computerized programs to treat anxiety. There are several such programs available (for recent reviews, see Cavanagh & Shapiro, 2004; Spek et al., 2006). The study also suggests it may be useful to prescreen patients for appropriateness for computerized CBT. Such triaging is consistent with a stepped-care approach in which patients with greater severity are referred directly to more intensive treatment. Consistent with our earlier discussion of financial barriers, an important lesson from this study is the importance of finding ways to make computerized CBT financially sustainable.

Self-help as an adjunct to standard psychotherapy

The two models described above suggest using self-help before entering face-to-face psychotherapy or concurrent with abbreviated face-to-face psychotherapy. However, self-help programs can be useful adjuncts to therapists providing standard 50-minute sessions of psychotherapy. In some cases, guides are available for clinicians on how to integrate self-help materials into treatment. For instance, there is a separate edition of *Mind Over Mood* to be used by clinicians (Padesky & Greenberger, 1995), and the MySelfHelp.com website includes a guide for helping clinicians match treatment goals with various modules in the web-based program (http://www.myselfhelp.com/Resources/Clinician_tips_DD.pdf).

As we discuss below, therapists may use self-help programs to provide psychoeducation or structure home practice of CBT skills, or as a resource for clients who are not receiving CBT for depression from their therapist. We should note that the feasibility of some of the strategies described below have not been formally evaluated in research. Nonetheless, we believe they reflect reasonable, incremental extensions of these empirically supported tools.

Self-help programs can assist in the provision of psychoeducation by assigning patients to complete modules that provide information about depression, as well as an introductory orientation to cognitive behavioral therapy (CBT). As noted previously, past studies have found that computer programs can be effective for enhancing knowledge about depression, decreasing stigma, and increasing literacy of CBT (Christensen et al., 2004; Wright et al., 2005). Clinicians can also make use of tools to assess patients' comprehension of self-help materials. Some web-based programs have self-scoring quizzes covering the content of the website. Scogin et al. (1998) developed a 23-item true-false test covering the content of *Feeling Good* (e.g. "Writing down your automatic negative thoughts will cause you to become more depressed."). At the end of each chapter of *Control Your Depression*, the authors present a checklist of review items to prompt readers to evaluate their comprehension (e.g. "I have learned to identify my non-constructive self-talk about difficult and unpleasant events."). Completing such quizzes or checklists before sessions can help structure the topics the patient wishes to address in the session.

Even if a clinician does not wish to use a computerized treatment program, web-based psychoeducation may be helpful. Patients with a variety of medical and psychiatric conditions are increasingly turning to the Internet for information; however, several studies have found that much of the information about depression online is not accurate and is potentially dangerous (Ernst & Schmidt, 2004; Griffiths & Christensen, 2000). We provide a list of several reputable websites to which patients may be referred (see Table 4.1).

A standard hallmark of CBT interventions is assigning between-session homework. There is some evidence that the more homework patients complete during CBT for depression, the more likely they are to achieve favorable treatment outcomes (Thase & Callen, 2006). Homework is thought of as a way to make the therapy session last all week and may include assigned readings, monitoring and challenging negative thoughts, or behavioral assignments to engage in positively reinforcing activities. In the final section of *The Feeling Good Handbook*, Burns (1999b) presents a chapter intended for therapists about how to introduce homework (referred to as "self-help") in treatment. This includes a memo that can be given to patients that introduces the idea of self-help as part of treatment and a list of activities that may constitute self-help, the majority of which involve activities for which structured instructions appear elsewhere in *Feeling Good*. A particularly creative hand-out includes a list of 24 reasons why people do not use self-help (e.g. perfectionistic thinking, fear of change, hopelessness) and asks patients to indicate the degree to which this issue may be influencing their resistance to make use of self-help. Such an assessment can provide useful guidance in terms of directing cognitive restructuring around maladaptive beliefs about self-help.

As noted above, books and computer programs can provide psychoeducation and orientation to CBT. Books and computer programs can also be used to introduce skills before a session so the therapist and patient can begin to apply the skill to a specific problem area earlier in the session. Exercises in books or standard modules of computerized psychotherapy could also be used to structure specific, therapist-designed homework assignments in cognitive restructuring, behavioral activation, or problem solving. The books described and most computer programs also include brief depression assessments that patients can use to self-monitor their symptoms. Patients could then bring their score and any automated feedback to the next session. In instances when sessions are spaced more than 1 week apart, clients could share assessment results with the clinician via email or telephone. Finally, as part of termination, a clinician may provide information about bibliotherapy or computerized treatment programs to be used for ongoing self-tracking of symptoms and as a resource for applying CBT to prevent relapse should symptoms re-emerge.

Because most book and computer programs apply CBT techniques, the most logical fit for using such programs is to augment a course of CBT for depression. However, a clinician may also choose to assign CBT self-help in situations when they are NOT providing CBT for depression in session but still feel that the client could benefit from exposure to CBT. There are at least three such scenarios. First, a therapist is using a specific CBT protocol to address a clinical problem that is comorbid with depression – for instance, exposure-based therapies for anxiety disorders – but still wishes to address depression simultaneously. Second, therapists may choose to use a different empirically supported therapeutic orientation to address depression in session – such as interpersonal therapy (Weissman et al., 2000) which is not available in a self-help format – but also wishes to also expose patients to some of the techniques of CBT. Third, some clinicians have not been trained in CBT or prefer a less-structured, eclectic, integrative, or supportive approach to therapy. With each of these scenarios, the clinician should use their best judgment as to whether combining approaches would be advantageous or overwhelming for a given client. Also, even if the clinician is not planning to use CBT for depression as the primary focus of therapy, they should still be familiar with the assigned book or computer programs and be prepared to discuss patient's questions about their content in session.

Integrated e-health systems for self-management and communication with clinicians

In the programs reviewed above, many integrate psychoeducation, assessment of symptoms, and psychotherapy. However, health care communication is increasingly conducted through electronic means. Patients routinely communicate with doctors via email. Electronic medical records facilitate the sharing of information among practitioners caring for the same patient. Integrated e-health systems hold the potential to further integrate the components of computerized psychoeducation, symptom monitoring, and psychotherapy with other electronic advances in health care communication. In a previous section, we discussed MySelfHelp.com, which includes options for users to share summaries of their site usage with clinicians. A program currently being developed by researchers in Perth, Western Australia called *RecoveryRoad* holds promise in this regard.

The program was described in a recent paper (Robertson et al., 2006). Patients currently being seen by a clinician were recruited to use the program as an adjunct to usual care. Patients were prompted via a reminder call to log onto the system for 12 sessions consisting of approximately 4 weekly sessions for the first month, 2 sessions the second month, 1 monthly session the third through sixth months, and 2 follow-up visits at months 9 and 12. At each visit, patients completed questionnaires assessing symptoms and medication adherence, and an automated report was generated and presented to the patient. The patient was then directed to additional resources, including psychoeducation, tips for overcoming depression, automated CBT, and an e-diary. Patients also maintained an online record of past and current medication. An innovative feature of this program is that patients can indicate which providers they would like to be able to access the information via the web, and clinicians can use the program to communicate with the patient or with other providers in the patient's treatment team. Patients control the privacy settings to determine which clinicians can access different information. Indicated clinicians can also be sent progress monitoring outcomes and flags to identify patients at risk.

In a recent pilot study (Robertson et al., 2006), 144 patients were referred to *RecoveryRoad* from various clinics in Perth, Western Australia. Adherence to the program was generally high, especially when patients received reminders from case workers (a feature added later in the study). Self-reported medication adherence was also higher in this group than for published norms. Patients using the program showed considerable improvement, but it is important to remember that all patients were receiving concurrent standard treatment from at least one provider. Future randomized control trials are needed to determine whether *RecoveryRoad* decreases depression symptoms above and beyond standard care. Nonetheless, both patients and clinicians reported high degrees of satisfaction with the program and the information it provided. Most relevant for the theme of self-management, all surveyed clinicians stated that this program helped patients to better manage their condition.

Dennis Tannenbaum, M.D., the creator of *RecoveryRoad*, indicates that the program continues to be refined (personal communication, August 2007). Recent evolutions include a non-CBT computerized psychotherapy focused more on illness adaptation and treatment compliance, greater use of case managers to monitor treatment and facilitate communication between providers, and customized programs for mild depression, chronic depression, and bipolar disorder.

Another promising program is LifeCoach, developed by LifeOptions, a Boston-based company that includes several specialty health care network and online media companies addressing the behavioral risks market (www2.lifeoptions.com). LifeCoach is not currently available directly to consumers but instead is purchased by employers and health care organizations, which in turn make the program available to employees and health plan subscribers. LifeCoach includes modules to address depression as well as other clinical issues, including insomnia, stress and anxiety, addictions, and trauma. A unique advantage of this application is that it is a scalable program that integrates the ideas of stepped-care with electronic communication between users and health care professionals. Visitors to the website first complete a standardized assessment and are then directed to an appropriate level of intervention based upon severity of symptoms. Interventions include web-based psychoeducation, paper bibliotherapy workbook resources, peer support message boards, and automated CBT-based programs. In addition, users can send a confidential email to a clinician, chat with one in real time using text messaging software, or speak with one on the phone. Clinician support is available 24 hours a day. The program also includes extensive multi-media content and self-assessments. Like MySelfHelp.com, no published studies of LifeCoach are currently available in peer-reviewed journals; however, this program also offers many more sophisticated features not available in the more widely researched programs reviewed earlier. As this newer generation of programs become more widely used, it is possible that more evidence of their efficacy will be published.

Summary and conclusions

Bibliotherapy and computerized psychotherapy hold promise for increasing access to psychotherapy and decreasing the cost of treating depression. Programs that provide information and specific coping strategies may be useful to patients in learning to self-manage depression. Research to date shows several programs are efficacious in reducing symptoms. Studies also suggest that treatment may be most feasible when integrated with some degree of clinician contact. We presented four models for integrating self-help into standard treatment for depression.

REFERENCES

Andersson G. Internet-based cognitive-behavioral self help for depression. *Expert Rev Neurother*. 2006; 6:1637–1642.

Andersson G, Bergstrom J, Hollandare F, Carlbring P, Kaldo V, Ekselius L. Internet-based self-help for depression: randomized controlled trial. *Br J Psychiatry*. 2005; 187:456–461.

Bower P, Gilbody S. Stepped care in psychological therapies: access, effectiveness and efficiency. Narrative literature review. *Br J Psychiatry*. 2005; 186(1):11–17.

Bowers W, Stuart S, MacFarlane R, Gorman L. Use of computer-administered cognitive-behavior therapy with depressed inpatients. *Depression*. 1993; 1:294–299.

Bright JI, Baker KD, Neimeyer RA. Professional and paraprofessional group treatments for depression: a comparison of cognitive-behavioral and mutual support interventions. *J Consult Clin Psychol*. 1999; 67(4):491–501.

Brown RA, Lewinsohn PM. A psychoeducational approach to the treatment of depression: comparison of group, individual, and minimal contact procedures. *J Consult Clin Psychol*. 1984; 52:774–783.

Burns DD. *Feeling Good*. New York: Signet; 1980.

Burns DD. *Feeling Good*. New York: Avon; 1999a.

Burns DD. *The Feeling Good Handbook*. New York: Plume; 1999b.

Cavanagh K, Shapiro DA. Computer treatment for common mental health problems. *J Clin Psychol*. 2004; 60:239–251.

Cavanagh K, Shapiro DA, van Den Berg S, Swain S, Barkham M, Proudfoot J. The effectiveness of computerized cognitive behavioural therapy in routine care. *Br J Clin Psychol*. 2006; 45:499–514.

Christensen H, Griffiths KM, Korten A. Web-based cognitive behavior therapy: analysis of site usage and changes in depression and anxiety scores. *J Med Internet Res*. 2002; 4:e3.

Christensen H, Griffiths KM, Jorm AF. Delivering interventions for depression by using the internet: randomized controlled trial. *Br Med J*. 2004; 328:265–269.

Christensen H, Griffiths KM, Mackinnon AJ, Brittliffe K. Online randomized controlled trial of brief and full cognitive behaviour therapy for depression. *Psychol Med*. 2006; 36:1737–1746.

Clarke G, Reid E, Eubanks D, O'Connor E, DeBar LL, Kelleher C, Lynch F, Nunley S. Overcoming depression on the internet (ODIN): a randomized controlled trial of an internet depression skills intervention program. *J Med Internet Res*. 2002; 4:e14.

Clarke G, Eubanks D, Reid E, Kelleher C, O'Connor E, DeBar LL, Lynch F, Nunley S, Gullion C. Overcoming depression on the internet (ODIN) (2): a randomized trial of a self-help depression skills program with reminders. *J Med Internet Res*. 2005; 7:e16.

Colby KM. A computer program using cognitive therapy to treat depressed patients. *Psychiatr Serv*. 1995; 46:1223–1225.

Cuijpers P. Bibliotherapy in unipolar depression: a meta-analysis. *J Behav Ther Exp Psychiatry*. 1997; 28:139–147.

Cuijpers P. A psychoeducational approach to the treatment of depression: a meta-analysis of Lewinsohn's "Coping With Depression" Course. *Behav Ther*. 1998; 29:521–533.

den Boer PCAM, Wiersma D, Van Den Bosch RJ. Why is self-help neglected in the treatment of emotional disorders? A meta-analysis. *Psychol Med*. 2004; 34:959–971.

Ernst E, Schmidt K. 'Alternative' cures for depression: how safe are web sites? *Psychiatry Res*. 2004; 129:297–301.

Floyd M, Scogin F, McKendree-Smith NL, Floyd DL, Rokke PD. Cognitive therapy for depression: a comparison of individual psychotherapy and bibliotherapy for depressed older adults. *Behav Modif*. 2004; 28:297–318.

Floyd M, Rohen N, Shackelford JAM, Hubbard KL, Parnell MB, Scogin F, Coates A. Two-year follow-up of bibliotherapy and individual cognitive therapy for depressed older adults. *Behav Modif*. 2006; 30:281–294.

Frankl V. *Man's Search for Meaning*. New York: Pocket Books; 1959.

Gega L, Marks I, Mataix-Cols D. Computer-aided CBT self-help for anxiety and depressive disorders: experience of a London clinic and future directions. *J Clin Psychol*. 2004; 60:147–157.

Graham C, Franses A, Kenwright M, Marks I. Problem severity in people using alternative therapies for anxiety difficulties. *Psychiatr Bull*. 2001; 25(1):12–14.

Gregory RJ, Schwer Canning S, Lee TW, Wise JC. Cognitive bibliotherapy for depression: a meta-analysis. *Prof Psychol Res Pr*. 2004; 35:275–280.

Griffiths KM, Christensen H. Quality of web based information on treatment of depression: cross sectional survey. *BMJ*. 2000; 321(7275):1511–1515.

Griffiths KM, Christensen H. Internet-based mental health programs: a powerful tool in the rural medical kit. *Aust J Rural Health*. 2007; 15:81–87.

Gum AM, Areán PA, Hunkeler E, Tang L, Katon W, Hitchcock, P, Steffens DC, Dickens J, Unützer J. Depression treatment preferences in older primary care patients. *Gerontologist*. 2006; 46:14–22.

Landreville P, Bissonnette L. Effects of cognitive bibliotherapy for depressed older adults with a disability. *Clin Gerontol*. 1997; 17:35–55.

Lewinsohn P, Muñoz R, Youngren MA, Zeiss A. *Control Your Depression*. Englewood Cliffs, NJ: Prentice Hall; 1978.

Lewinsohn P, Muñoz R, Breckenridge JS, Zeiss A. The *"Coping with Depression" Course*. Eugene, OR: Castila; 1984.

Lewinsohn P, Muñoz R, Youngren MA, Zeiss A. Control Your Depression: Revised Edition. New York, NY: Fireside; 1992.

Lamberg L. On-line empathy for mood disorders: patients turn to internet support groups. *J Am Med Assoc*. 2003; 289:3073–3077.

Macdonald W, Mead N, Bower P, Richards D, Lovell K. A qualitative study of patients' perceptions of a 'minimal' psychological therapy. *Int J Soc Psychiatry*. 2007; 53(1):23–35.

Mahalik JR, Kivlighan DM Jr. Self-help treatment for depression: who succeeds? *J Couns Psychol*. 1988; 35:237–242.

Mains JA, Scogin FR. The effectiveness of self-administered treatments: a practice-friendly review of the research. *J Clin Psychol*. 2003; 59(2):237–246.

Marks IM, Mataix-Cols D, Kenwright M, Cameron R, Hirsch S, Gega L. Pragmatic evaluation of computer-aided self-help for anxiety and depression. *Br J Psychiatry*. 2003; 183:57–65.

Marrs RW. A meta-analysis of bibliotherapy studies. *Am J Community Psychol*. 1995; 23(6):843–870.

McCrone P, Knapp M, Proudfoot J, Ryden C, Cavanagh K, Shapiro DA, Ilson S, Gray JA, Goldberg D, Mann A, Marks I, Everitt B, Tylee A. Cost-effectiveness of computerized cognitive-behavioural therapy for anxiety and depression in primary care: randomized controlled trial. *Br J Psychiatry*. 2004; 185:55–62.

National Institute for Health and Clinical Excellence. *Computerised cognitive behaviour therapy for depression and anxiety*. 2006. Available at http://www.nice.org.uk/nicemedia/pdf/TA097guidance.pdf. Retrieved on July 24, 2008.

Norcross JC. Here comes the self-help revolution in mental heath. *Psychother Theory Res Pract Training*. 2000; 37(4):370–377.

Norcross JC. Integrating self-help into psychotherapy: 16 practical suggestions. *Prof Psychol Res Pr.* 2006; 37(6):683–693.

Osgood-Hynes DJ, Greist JH, Marks IM, Baer L, Heneman SW, Wenzel KW, Manzo PA, Parkin JR, Spierings CJ, Dottl SL, Vitse HM. Self-administered psychotherapy for depression using a telephone-accessed computer system plus booklets: an open U.S.-U.K. study. *J Clin Psychiatry.* 1998; 59:358–365.

Padesky CA, Greenberger D. *Clinician's Guide to "Mind Over Mood."* New York, NY: Guilford Press; 1995.

Patten SB. Prevention of depressive symptoms through the use of distance technologies. *Psychiatr Serv.* 2003; 54:396–398.

Pew Internet and American Life Project. Internet health resources. 2003. Available at http://www.pewinternet.org/pdfs/pip_health_report_july_2003.pdf. Retrieved July 24, 2008.

Proudfoot J, Goldberg D, Mann A, Everitt B, Marks I, Gray JA. Computerized, interactive, multimedia cognitive-behavioural program for anxiety and depression in general practice. *Psychol Med.* 2003; 33:217–227.

Proudfoot J, Ryden C, Everitt B, Shapiro DA, Goldberg D, Mann A, Tylee A, Marks I, Gray JA. Clinical efficacy of computerized cognitive-behavioural therapy for anxiety and depression in primary care: randomized controlled trial. *Br J Psychiatry.* 2004; 185:46–54.

Redding RE, Herbert JD, Forman EM, Gaudiano BA. Popular self-help books for anxiety, depression, and trauma: how scientifically grounded and useful are they? *Prof Psychol Res Pr.* 2008; 39:537–545.

Robertson L, Smith M, Castle D, Tannenbaum D. Using the Internet to enhance the treatment of depression. *Australas Psychiatry.* 2006; 14(4):413–417.

Rosen GM. Self-help treatment books and the commercialization of psychotherapy. *Am Psychol.* 1987; 42(1):46–51.

Rosen GM. Self-help or hype? Comments on psychology's failure to advance self-care. *Prof Psychol Res Practice.* 1993; 24:340–345.

Schmidt MM, Miller WR. Amount of therapist contact and outcome in multi-dimensional depression treatment program. *Acta Psychiatr Scand.* 1983; 67:319–332.

Scogin F, Hamblin D, Beutler L. Bibliotherapy for depressed older adults: a self-help alternative. *Gerontologist.* 1987; 27:383–387.

Scogin F, Jamison C, Gochneur K. Comparative efficacy of cognitive and behavioral bibliotherapy for mildly and moderately depressed older adults. *J Consult Clin Psychol.* 1989; 57:403–407.

Scogin F, Jamison C, Davis N. Two-year follow-up of bibliotherapy for depression in older adults. *J Consult Clin Psychol.* 1990; 58:665–667.

Scogin F, Jamison C, Floyd M, Chaplin WF. Measuring learning in depression treatment: a cognitive bibliotherapy test. *Cognit Ther Res.* 1998; 22(5):475–482.

Scogin FR, Hanson A, Welsh D. Self-administered treatment in stepped-care models of depression treatment. *J Clin Psychol.* 2003; 59(3):341–349.

Selmi PM, Klein MH, Greist JH, Sorrell SP, Erdman HP. Computer-administered cognitive-behavioral therapy for depression. *Am J Psychiatry.* 1990; 147:51–56.

Sirovatka P. Hyman leaves NIMH stronger, richer. *Psychiatr Res Rep.* 2002; 18:2.

Slack W V. *Cybermedicine: How Computing Empowers Doctors and Patients for Better Health Care*. Rev. and updated edn. San Francisco, CA: Jossey-Bass; 2001.

Spek V, Cuijpers P, Nyklicek I, Riper H, Keyzer J, Pop V. Internet-based cognitive behaviour therapy for symptoms of depression and anxiety: a meta-analysis. *Psychol Med*. 2006; 37:1797–1806.

Stutzke T, Aiken L, Stout C. Maximizing treatment outcome in managed care: useful technological adjunct. *Independent Pract*. 1997; 17:27–29.

Thase ME, Callan JA. The role of homework in cognitive behavior therapy of depression. *J Psychother Integration*. 2006; 16:162–177.

van Den Berg S, Shapiro DA, Bickerstaffe D, Cavanagh K. Computerized cognitive-behaviour therapy for anxiety and depression: a practical solution to the shortage of trained therapists. *J Psychiatr Ment Health Nurs*. 2004; 11:508–513.

Vos T, Corry J, Haby MM, Carter R, Andrews G. Cost-effectiveness of cognitive-behavioural therapy and drug interventions for major depression. *Aust N Z J Psychiatry*. 2005; 39(8):683–692.

Walker JR, Vincent N, Furor P. Self-help treatments for anxiety disorders. In Antony MM, Stein MB, eds: *Oxford Handbook of Anxiety and Related Disorders*. New York: Oxford University Press; 2009, pp 488–496.

Weissman M M, Markowitz JC, Klerman GL. *Comprehensive Guide to Interpersonal Psychotherapy*. New York, NY: Basic Books; 2000.

Whitfield G, Hinshelwood R, Pashely A, Campshie L, Williams C. The impact of a novel computerized CBT CD Rom (Overcoming Depression) offered to patients referred to clinical psychology. *Behav Cognit Psychother*. 2005; 34:1–11.

Whitfield G, Williams CJ, Shapiro DA. Assessing the take up and acceptability of a self-help room used by patients awaiting their initial outpatient appointment. *Behav Cognit Psychother*. 2001; 29:333–343.

Wollersheim JP, Wilson GL. Group treatment of unipolar depression: a comparison of coping, supportive, bibliotherapy and delayed treatment groups. *Prof Psychol Res Pract*. 1991; 22:496–502.

Wright JH, Wright AS, Albano AM, Basco MR, Goldsmith LJ, Raffield T, Otto, MW. Computer-assisted cognitive therapy for depression: maintaining efficacy while reducing therapist time. *Am J Psychiatry*. 2005; 162:1158–1164.

Physical exercise as a form of self-management for depression

The benefits of exercise for physical health are beyond dispute. Exercise is also held in high esteem as a treatment for depression. As many as 85% of physicians view exercise as a valid treatment for depression (Dishman, 1986). Psychotherapists providing cognitive behavioral therapy (CBT) also frequently emphasize increasing physical activity as a treatment goal. Patients in one study receiving a comprehensive psychiatric treatment program that includes exercises indicated that exercise was the most important component (Martinsen, 1990). Patients may also view exercise as a common sense, non-pharmacological, non-stigmatizing approach to depression treatment. As will be seen in this chapter, aerobic and non-aerobic forms of exercise have been shown to be an efficacious treatment for depression in over 25 years of research.

Exercise is also highly consistent with the qualities of depression self-management strategies outlined in Chapter 1. Exercise is practiced outside of the context of face-to-face interactions with primary care or mental health providers and can be effectively overseen by care managers or paraprofessionals. Exercise can be self-titrated by a patient to regulate mood or other symptoms of depression. As such, it empowers patients to take a more active role in managing their depression. After successful treatment, exercise has the potential to be an enduring strategy that patients retain in their "toolkits" for use as a relapse prevention strategy. Although exercise is a promising form of self-management, most patients will require some support and guidance from treatment providers to implement and sustain a program of exercise.

Many clinicians reading this introduction are likely aware of the promise of exercise. However, they likely have also had the experience of recommending or prescribing exercise to a depressed patient and being disappointed with that patient's adherence. They may feel that exercise works under controlled conditions of research studies, but doesn't work as well in their practice with their patients. After critically reviewing the research to date and discussing potential limitations in generalizability of findings, we present practical recommendations for clinicians interested in incorporating physical exercise into their treatment plans for patients with depression. Along with guidance in specifics of incorporating exercise into a treatment program, we provide practical suggestions for enhancing patient motivation and optimizing adherence.

Research on exercise as a treatment for depression

History and summary of studies

Exercise encompasses a variety of planned or structured physical activity undertaken to improve aerobic fitness, strength, endurance, flexibility, or body composition. In the past 30 years, research on the link between exercise and depression has grown steadily. In 1984, it was estimated that over 1000 studies had been published on the relationship between exercise and mood (Hughes, 1984) and this number has likely doubled since that time. Not all of these studies are of high-quality or speak directly to the relationship between exercise and clinical depression. Nonetheless, interest in this area has continued to grow, with researchers employing increasing methodological sophistication and rigor. A variety of correlational studies have shown intriguing links between physical fitness, activity levels, and depression. Early research found that individuals with depression had poorer muscular endurance than non-depressed controls and, among hospitalized depressed patients, poorer grip strength and muscular endurance at intake predicted longer hospitalizations (Morgan, 1968). Contemporary, population-based studies have documented that sedentary lifestyle is associated with depression symptom severity and likelihood of diagnoses of major depressive disorder (MDD) (see Biddle, 2000; and Stathopoulou et al., 2006 for summaries and reviews of this literature).

Studies of exercise as a treatment for clinical depression emerged in the late 1970s and early 1980s. In one of the earliest published studies, Greist and collaborators (1979) found that 8 patients assigned to begin a program of running showed symptom improvements comparable to a group of 15 patients receiving psychotherapy. In the years since this pilot study was published, many large-scale, randomized controlled studies have been conducted, focusing mainly on aerobic exercise including walking and jogging and non-aerobic resistance training. Two recent meta-analyses provide estimates of the effects of exercise on depression relative to inactive control conditions such as waitlists or health education classes. Lawlor and Hopker (2001) analyzed 11 studies where patients diagnosed with depression were randomized to receive either exercise or a control condition. More recently, Stathopoulou and colleagues (2006) updated the Lawlor and Hopker (2001) meta-analysis by including four subsequently published studies and excluding studies not published in peer-reviewed journals and those in which participants had subclinical levels of depression. Compared with inactive comparison conditions, exercise produced a large effect in reducing depression scores in both reviews. Stathopoulou and colleagues

(2006) estimated that it would require 367 unpublished or future studies finding no effect for exercise to negate the effects of the 11 studies included in their meta-analysis.

Taken together, these studies help to rule out spontaneous remission as an explanation for improvements during exercise. They also suggest that exercising is vastly superior to receiving no treatment for depression. An important question is whether exercise is comparable to established treatments for depression. One study found no difference in degree of improvement among individuals assigned to individual cognitive therapy alone, exercise alone, or combination of exercise and cognitive therapy (Fremont & Craighead, 1987). Lawlor and Hopker (2001) identified three other studies that also failed to find significant differences between exercise and cognitive therapy; however, it should be noted that two of these studies are unpublished doctoral dissertations. Exercise has also been shown to be equally effective as antidepressant medication. In this widely cited study, Blumenthal and colleagues (1999) randomized 156 older adults with major depressive disorder (MDD) to one of three conditions: a 4-month trial of either medication (sertraline), aerobic exercise, or a combination of medication and exercise. At the end of the study, all three conditions experienced clinically significant improvement in depression; however, none of the conditions proved to be superior at the end of the 4 months.

Given that exercise is clearly superior to no treatment and appears to be comparably efficacious to standard treatments, several recent studies are working to identify the optimal "dose" of exercise for treating depression. One study (Dunn et al., 2005) randomized 80 participants to one of three conditions: the consensus public health recommended dose of weekly energy expenditure on a treadmill or stationary bicycle (17.5 kcal/kg/week), a lower dose of energy expenditure using similar equipment (7.0 kcal/kg/week), and an exercise placebo group consisting of stretching exercises. The public health dosage was found to be more effective than the lower dosage, which performed similarly to placebo (flexibility exercises). Interestingly, frequency of exercise was less of a factor than dosage; it did not appear to matter if either weekly dosage was spread out over 3 or 5 days. A dose-response study of non-aerobic exercise (Singh et al., 2005) randomized participants to weightlifting at high intensity (80% of their one-repetition maximum capacity), weightlifting at low intensity (20% capacity), or standard care by a primary care physician. The high-intensity group had nearly double the response rate of participants in either the low-intensity or standard care conditions. Taken together, these results suggest that higher dosages of exercise may produce greater reductions in depression symptoms.

Populations

Exercise interventions have been shown to be efficacious in a variety of adult populations. Studies have generally focused on individuals with mild to moderate levels of depression. The most common age groups for inclusion in studies have been elderly, middle-aged adults, and college students. In general, there is currently little evidence in support of exercise as an effective treatment for children and adolescents with depression; however, most studies to date have considerable methodological limitations (Larun et al., 2006). Exercise has also been found to be efficacious in several specialty populations, including women with post-partum depression (Armstrong & Edwards, 2004), inpatients (Sexton et al., 1989; Bosscher, 1993), and patients who have failed to fully respond to antidepressant medication (Mather et al., 2002; Trivedi et al., 2006).

Potential mechanisms

Several biological and psychological hypotheses have been presented for the antidepressant properties of exercise. One hypothesis building largely on animal studies of exercise posits that exercise leads to neurogenesis in the hippocampus comparable to changes observed in human patients following treatment with antidepressants and electroconvulsive therapy (Ernst et al., 2006). Other biological theories have focused on exercise's proposed role in the modification of serotonin function and the release of endorphins. These studies are based largely on laboratory neuroendocrine challenge paradigms comparing sedentary and physically active adults (for a summary, see Stathopoulou et al., 2006). Other findings suggest alternate biological pathways. including reducing hypothalamic-pituitary-adrenal (HPA) axis activity (Van Der Pompe et al., 1999) and inflammatory processes (Smith, 2006), increasing aerobic capacity (Blumenthal et al., 1999) and physical strength (Singh et al., 2005), improving sleep quality (Singh et al., 1997; Singh et al., 2005), and regulation of activity in the prefrontal cortex as measured by tasks assessing executive functioning (Kubesch et al., 2003).

Several psychological theories have also been applied and received some research support. Consistent with a cognitive model of depression treatment, initiating and maintaining an exercise program may help boost feelings of mastery, self-efficacy, and self-esteem (Blumenthal et al., 1999; Craft, 2005). In keeping with models of depression emphasizing behavioral and emotion regulation factors, exercise has the potential to be a form of behavioral activation in that it reduces the depressive action tendencies of avoidance and withdrawal and, instead, puts an individual in contact with rewarding environments (Dimidjian et al., 2006; Hopko et al., 2003; Stathopoulou et al., 2006). From a behavioral perspective, energy gains associated with enhanced physical fitness may lead the patient to make changes in their environment; namely, increasing engagement with pleasant activities and reducing stress through more active coping. Also in keeping with emotion regulation perspectives, individuals in exercise programs have been shown to decrease ruminative thinking and increase their use of adaptive mental distraction from depressive thoughts (Craft, 2005; Hughes, 1984).

Adding to the challenge of identifying pathways is disentangling the complex integration of biological and psychological factors. Mechanisms of the antidepressant effect of exercise are an ongoing area of research. Nonetheless, the biological and psychosocial models based on existing research provide clinicians with a range of rationales to present to patients when encouraging them to exercise.

Summary

Exercise has been shown to be superior to no treatment, the efficacy is comparable to established treatment, and these findings have been replicated across multiple research groups. Thus physical exercise satisfies several of the key criteria of a "well-established," empirically supported psychosocial treatment, as defined by the American Psychological Association's Task Force for Promotion and Dissemination of Psychological Procedures (Chambless & Hollon, 1998). It has been shown to be effective in a variety of depressed adult populations, and several potential mechanisms have been identified. However, important limitations are present in nearly all of the clinical trials reviewed earlier (Lawlor & Hopker, 2001; Sjösten & Kivelä, 2006). These limitations will be discussed in the following section.

Critiques and remaining questions from exercise treatment studies

Although their meta-analysis found a large effect for exercise as a treatment for depression, Lawlor and Hopker (2001) stated that, due to methodological problems in the studies reviewed, it was not possible to determine whether exercise truly is an efficacious treatment for depression. The magnitude of observed effects can be inflated by several common problems in many of these studies, including inadequate concealment of randomization, limited reporting of intent-to-treat analyses, and non-blinded assessments (Lawlor and Hopker, 2001; Sjösten & Kivelä, 2006). Many of these methodological limitations – which are present in other early depression treatment literature – are increasingly being addressed in more recent studies. In the following sections, we will focus on four questions about this literature: (1) Do treatment effects continue to last after the structured intervention? (2) When exercise is added to medication or psychotherapy, does it produce more improvement than either approach alone? (3) Can findings generalize to patients outside of research studies? (4) Is social contact a better explanation for why people improve with depression treatment? These issues present important limitations and caveats that may inform how research findings are translated into clinical implementation of exercise as a self-management strategy.

Durability of the effects of exercise

Lawlor and Hopker (2001) noted that many studies available when they conducted their meta-analyses failed to report long-term efficacy data. A particularly troubling counterintuitive finding from the Lawlor and Hopker (2001) review was that exercise programs with longer duration (greater than 8 weeks) tended to show weaker effects than shorter trials (less than 8 weeks). The authors interpret this to suggest "the effects may be sustained only in the short term." This conclusion reaches somewhat beyond the data in that patients were not randomized to programs of differing duration, and symptom trajectories were not systematically analyzed to test for the hypothesized loss of treatment efficacy. This critique must also be considered in the context of recent findings that the durability of the benefits from treatment with antidepressants is also quite modest (Rush et al., 2006). Nonetheless, the question of the durability of findings remained ambiguous at the time of this review.

Since the Lawlor and Hopker (2001) review was published, newer studies with systematic follow-up data paint a more hopeful picture. In a sample of elderly patients with major or minor depressive disorder randomized to either progressive resistance training (i.e. weightlifting) or attentional control, the exercise group showed greater improvement in depression both at the end of the 20-week study period and at the 26-month follow-up (Singh et al., 1997; Singh et al., 2001). Two years later, a third of this group was still engaging in regular weightlifting. In contrast, a second study of geriatric patients with poorly responsive depressive disorder randomized to either 10 weeks of exercise classes or health education talks (i.e. the control condition) found no advantage for exercise classes 24 weeks after the intervention had ended (Mather et al., 2002). However, it should be noted that only modest differences in depression scores were found at the end of the 10-week intervention, and the authors did not indicate the degree to which participants continued with regular exercise after the classes ended.

One of the most intriguing patterns of follow-up results came from the Blumenthal and colleagues' (1999) study of older adults described earlier. As noted previously, at the end of 4 months of treatment, the exercise-only group showed comparable gains to the medication-only and medication plus exercise conditions at the end. However, 6 months after structured treatment ended, a somewhat different story emerged. Based on rates of remission derived from clinician interviews, significantly more of the patients in the exercise group had achieved remission than either the medication-only group or the medication plus exercise groups (Babyak et al., 2000). This finding is remarkable in that it is perhaps the only study to demonstrate superiority of exercise (instead of equivalence) to established treatments.

Furthermore, significantly fewer of the remitted participants in the exercise condition had relapsed relative to either of the conditions including medication

(Babyak et al., 2000). This finding suggests that exercise may have important relapse prevention properties. The authors were surprised by the superiority of the exercise condition over the medication plus exercise condition. Qualitatively, the authors noted a strong "anti-medication" sentiment among some of the participants randomized to conditions involving medication, although this was not systematically measured in their study. This potential alternative explanation, as well as side effects of medication, should be explored in future studies; however, it speaks to a clinical reality that many patients with depression would prefer a non-pharmacological approach to treating their symptoms. These patients may be more committed to achieving benefits when offered such an approach.

The superior outcomes in the exercise-only condition of this study were especially true among patients who had continued exercising during the 6-month period that followed the initial 4-month treatment. This is consistent with Martinsen (1990), who reported that depressed patients who continued to exercise in the year following training programs tended to have lower depression scores than those who became sedentary.

Taken together, results of newer studies suggest that antidepressant effects of exercise can be durable in the long term and may have relapse prevention properties. However, having patients remain physically active may be a key factor in maintaining these treatment gains. Although some of the concerns raised by Lawlor and Hopker (2001) have been addressed by newer studies, it is important that future trials continue to examine both durability of effects and the degree of maintenance of exercise following structured treatment programs.

Incremental value of adding exercise to established treatment

Many studies have examined exercise as a monotherapy; however, fewer have examined whether adding exercise to another form of treatment has any incremental efficacy above and beyond the original treatment. An early study of inpatients with MDD receiving non-specific psychotherapy and in some cases medication (tricyclic antidepressants) found that those randomized to an aerobic exercise as an adjunctive treatment showed greater improvement than those randomized to a control group (Martinsen et al., 1985), who continued to receive only standard care. A later randomized trial found some additional benefits to adding aerobic exercise to standard care (Veale et al., 1992). As noted previously, in a randomized trial, Blumenthal et al. (1999) found no relative advantage to combining exercise and medication (sertraline) at the end of 4 months of treatment relative to either approach as a monotherapy. Paradoxically, the combined treatment led to higher relapse rates than exercise alone 6 months after treatment ended. Although this result has yet to be replicated, it suggests that combining treatments may actually be contraindicated. In contrast, a randomized control trial by Mather et al. (2002) found that adding weight-bearing exercise to outpatient pharmacotherapy produced higher rates of response than a control condition of health education talks. As Stathopoulou et al. (2006) note, few studies of exercise as an adjunct to cognitive therapy have been conducted, although the one existing study failed to show an advantage (Fremont & Craighead, 1987).

The limited advantages of combining exercise with other treatments echo the relatively limited added benefit of combining cognitive behavioral therapy (CBT) and medication in mild to moderate depression (Feldman, 2007). In the case of CBT and medication, advantages of combination therapies are usually more robust in patients with more chronic or severe forms of depression, a group not typically studied in exercise intervention research. A similar pattern may be true with regard to combining exercise with medication or psychotherapy. This is an important question for future research. Taken together, results at this point are mixed regarding the incremental benefits of combining exercise and medication, especially when exercise and the second treatment are started simultaneously.

A promising future direction for research is the use of exercise as an augmentation strategy to antidepressant medication, that is, an adjunctive therapy for those who have at least some residual symptoms following an initial course of antidepressant medication (Trivedi et al., 2006). In the Mather et al. (2002) study described earlier, an inclusion criterion was failure to respond to adequate dose of antidepressants after at least a 6-week trial. In a recent open-trial pilot study, 17 patients with incomplete remission from antidepressant medication were assigned to a 12-week customized exercise program (Trivedi et al., 2006). Overall, patients showed significant improvement. However, these results are preliminary and need to be supported with a controlled trial. Nonetheless, it suggests that a sequenced approach may be most effective. It could be that when patients have partially recovered, they are more likely to engage with an exercise program. It is also possible that the demands of beginning two new treatments simultaneously may be overwhelming for a patient, thus reducing the degree of benefit from either treatment.

Generalizability

Clinicians reading these reviews may be eager to know to what degree these results are generalizable to the patients they work with in their clinics. Two issues are worthy of review. First is the manner in which patients were recruited and the severity of their symptoms.

Lawlor & Hopker (2001) note that many studies relied on community volunteer samples rather than clinically referred patients. Such patients may be more motivated, active, and potentially less severe than clinically referred patients, thus potentially skewing the findings. It is worth mentioning that several studies have included inpatient samples and physician-referred patients who may more closely resemble typical clinic patients. Nonetheless, patients in these studies would have been informed that exercise was one of the possible conditions in the study and patients who would have been physically unable to comply with an exercise program or unwilling to commit to trying it would likely have been screened out.

Some clinicians may wonder whether studies are biased by inclusion of less severe populations. Indeed, some exercise treatment studies have used samples with subclinical symptom severity. However, it is worth remembering that a large effect was found in the Stathopoulou et al. (2006) meta-analysis which excluded studies using participants with subclinical levels of depression. On average, participants in these studies were in the moderate range of severity. It should also be noted that degree of severity at baseline was not found to be associated with magnitude of effect sizes in the Lawlor and Hopker (2001) review. In other words, studies with more severe populations did not systematically show less improvement. Therefore, results do not appear to be biased by severity within the mild to moderate range. Patients with severe depression have not been typically studied; thus clinicians working with this population would be encouraged to follow treatment guidelines and use antidepressant medication and/or an empirically supported form of psychotherapy as a first-line treatment. Exercise may be a fruitful adjunctive treatment after a sufficient trial of medication has been initiated.

Is social contact a better explanation for the effects of exercise?

Another important caveat of past studies is that nearly all involved some form of social contact. Many studies had participants exercise in groups, and nearly all involved contact with trainers who supervised some aspect of the exercise. This issue is particularly important in studies where group exercise was compared with an individually administered treatment, such as pharmacotherapy in the Blumenthal et al. (1999) study. Newer studies have been more sensitive to this potential confound and have had participants exercise individually (Dunn et al., 2005, Singh et al., 2005), although this still involved some contact with a supervising trainer. One study of moderately depressed, community-dwelling older adults is particularly telling in this regard (McNeil et al., 1991). Participants were randomized to either three weekly walking sessions accompanied by an undergraduate psychology student instructed to engage the participant in casual conversation or two weekly visits from a student who was similarly instructed to engage the participant in conversation. Both groups showed comparable improvement relative to a control condition, but exercise plus social contact was not found to be superior to social contact alone. However, recent studies found that exercise was superior to social control conditions including health education classes (Mather et al., 2002; Singh et al., 1997). Similarly, another study found that participating in group "pram-walking" (i.e. walking while pushing a baby carriage or stroller) was more effective at reducing symptoms of post-partum depression than was participation in an unstructured playgroup (Armstrong & Edwards, 2004).

Studies of group exercise that do not control for social contact are left with this potential confound that may account in part for the effects observed. Given the potential importance of contact with either other patients or supervising trainers, in our section on clinical recommendations, we will discuss strategies for optimizing exercise programs by building in external structure and social contact.

Challenges in implementing exercise as a treatment for depression

As a clinical population, patients with depression may reflect a particularly challenging group to engage with exercise. Depression itself is characterized by apathy, pessimism, and deficits in physical energy and self-confidence. Problem-solving may be especially challenging for patients with depression, either due to state-dependent difficulties with effortful cognition, underlying deficits in problem-solving skills, or some combination. Furthermore, some patients with depression may have a low frustration tolerance and have difficulty rebounding from initial setbacks in an exercise program (Seime & Vickers, 2006). Patients with depression are more likely to be physically sedentary and have a reduced work capacity relative to the general population (Martinsen, 1990). Each of these deficits may undermine a patient's ability to initiate or persist with an exercise program.

Adherence is an important concern in exercise programs generally. Past studies suggest that one in four individuals do not adhere to short-term prescribed exercise, and after 6 months, two in four do not adhere (Stathopoulou et al., 2006). Rates of adherence could be expected to be even lower in depressed populations due to the motivational and self-regulation deficits described in the previous paragraph (Seime & Vickers, 2006). In research studies, attrition from exercise programs is generally modest and comparable to pharmacotherapy treatment studies for depression. Estimates from the Stathopoulou et al. (2006) meta-analysis suggest that roughly one in five patients will drop out of exercise treatment. As discussed earlier, it is worth remembering that samples in exercise studies may reflect a self-selection bias and thus optimal adherence for depressed patients. Also, nearly all of the studies in the Stathopoulou et al. (2006) review provided participants with ongoing supervision. When supervised exercise terminates, rates of continued adherence range from 64% at 6 months (Babyak et al., 2000) to 33% at 26 months (Singh et al., 2001). One recent pilot study which initiated 9 weeks of independent exercise after 3 weeks of supervised intervention found that of the 17 participants enrolled in the study, only 8 completed the program (Trivedi et al. 2006). These findings clearly highlight the challenge of having patients with depression maintain exercise outside of supervised settings.

Is there any way of knowing in advance which patients with depression are most likely to fail to maintain an exercise program? Although there is little formal research into situational or patient factors predicting drop-out, some patterns do emerge when comparing studies with extremely high and low levels of attrition. Three studies of patients assigned to weightlifting and walking had practically zero attrition (McNeil et al., 1991; Singh et al., 1997; Singh et al., 2005) compared with three studies of jogging and running, where drop-out was roughly 40% (Doyne et al., 1987; Klein et al., 1985; Sexton et al., 1989). Although there are many factors that differentiate the samples and study conditions across these six studies, it is possible that the higher level of exertion required by running and jogging discouraged some participants.

Data from the Blumenthal study, in which the drop-out rate was typical at 21%, were examined to identify individual differences that predicted drop-out (Herman et al., 2002). Higher levels of anxiety and lower levels of life satisfaction at baseline were the strongest predictors of treatment drop-out across all three conditions (exercise alone, pharmacotherapy alone, pharmacotherapy plus exercise). This suggests possible subgroups that may require additional support to remain with treatment. Interestingly, a counterintuitive finding was that higher physical symptoms at baseline actually predicted less drop-out in the exercise-only condition. This suggests that, among patients healthy enough to participate in an exercise program, those with some physical complaints may be more motivated to persist with exercise, perhaps because they are hopeful that it will relieve these somatic complaints (Herman et al., 2002).

Practical recommendations for incorporating exercise into a treatment plan

As we have reviewed in the preceding sections, exercise shows considerable promise as a treatment for depression and as a potential form of self-management. However, as we discussed, studies may provide an optimistic estimate of adherence given the self-selected nature of participants. Furthermore, the symptoms of depression and its associated psychopathology in self-regulation may place patients at a distinct disadvantage in beginning and monitoring an exercise program. In the following section, we discuss practical recommendations for integrating exercise into a treatment program with an eye towards addressing barriers that may interfere with treatment adherence. This section is divided into three sections. The first section reviews initial decisions providers should make about to whom they may wish to recommend exercise and what role they wish to play in supervising the exercise program. The second section focuses on the content of an exercise training program in terms of customizing type and dosages of exercise and the use of supporting structures to optimize success. The third section addresses how to enhance a patient's motivation for commencing and maintaining an exercise program and strategies for addressing non-adherence.

Initial decisions

To whom should exercise be recommended?

The first question that should guide such a decision is safety. Does the patient have any physical health concerns that preclude some form of exercise? As such, it would be appropriate to screen for relevant cardiovascular, immunological, and joint and muscle conditions that may rule out some or all forms of exercise. Such information would be known to a primary care physician but may not be part of a standard intake interview in mental health settings. A useful screening tool, the Physical Activity Readiness Questionnaire (PAR-Q), has been developed by the Canadian Society for Exercise Physiology and is available for download and use free of charge (www.csep.ca/forms.asp). If a mental health clinician has any question about the safety of initiating an exercise program for a given patient, consultation with the patient's physician is indicated. Such inquiry is an excellent opportunity to open the door to further collaboration between the mental health professional and the primary care doctor (Stathopoulou et al., 2006). As we will discuss in a later section, it is possible that in patients for whom aerobic exercise is contraindicated, non-aerobic exercise may be a viable alternative, which has also been shown to produce relief of depression symptoms. Exercise can be safely combined with serotonin reuptake inhibitors, the most commonly prescribed antidepressant.

Assuming that a patient is physically able to engage in exercise, is there an ideal patient to whom exercise should be recommended? As noted previously, depressed patients with high anxiety symptoms and lower life satisfaction may be less likely to remain with or benefit from an exercise treatment (Herman et al., 2002). Furthermore, it is likely to be most successful with patients who are reasonably motivated to try an exercise program. That said, in a later section, we will discuss strategies for enhancing motivation in patients who may be ambivalent about beginning an exercise program.

The other factor in treatment planning concerns when to use exercise as a first-line approach or in combination with other treatment modalities. Antidepressant medication and cognitive behavioral therapy (CBT) are typical first-line treatments for mild to moderate depression. However, given that exercise has been found to be similarly efficacious in head-to-head comparisons with medication or cognitive therapy, it is worth considering exercise as a first-line treatment in patients for whom medication or psychotherapy may not be appropriate. Exercise may be a more preferable treatment than medication among patients who are pregnant, breast-feeding, opposed to taking medication, or unable to tolerate side effects. Exercise may be preferable to psychotherapy for patients who are uncomfortable or unwilling to discuss the more emotional and interpersonal aspects of their experience of depression due to cultural norms or personal preference (Smith, 2006). Exercise may be an ideal behavioral intervention in situations where access to empirically supported psychotherapy may be limited due to geographic regions or long waitlists.

For all other patients, the combination of exercise with another form of treatment would be the most conservative route. As noted previously, there is some evidence that commencing exercise concurrently with another established treatment has little incremental advantage (Blumenthal et al., 1999; Fremont & Craighead, 1987). Instead, in combination treatments, it may be useful to begin exercise as an augmentation strategy for partial responders (Mather et al., 2002; Trivedi et al., 2006).

Decide on the clinician's role

Depending on their role in a patient's treatment team, clinicians will differ as to the degree to which they will be involved in structuring and monitoring their patient's exercise program. For instance, beginning a program of exercise would be a goal entirely consistent with the principle of behavioral activation in CBT for depression. Furthermore, assigning outside-of-session "homework," such as exercise and the types of cognitive, motivational, goal-setting, and problem-solving interventions described in more detail below, fit nicely within the repertoire of interventions of CBT. Thus exercise could be easily woven into a treatment plan. For clinicians interested in designing the specifics of an exercise treatment program with patients, we present specific guidelines in the next section.

On the other hand, for the primary care physician who has less contact with a patient and is managing all other medical systems, it may be more feasible to make a referral to a qualified personal trainer or other exercise or sports-medicine professional as an adjunctive treatment (Stathopoulou et al., 2006). Even in settings such as cognitive behavioral psychotherapy, it is possible that other issues may be a higher priority for in-session attention. We discuss the use of personal trainers in a later section. At a minimum, the clinician recommending exercise should inquire about the exercise program at each visit, offer to troubleshoot obstacles to adherence, and provide positive reinforcement for any efforts made.

What to recommend

When recommending that a patient begin exercising, it is important that a clinician work with the patient to develop a customized, specific, and realistic program of exercise. In this section, we discuss assessment strategies, guidelines, and tools that will assist in planning a treatment program. Based on a review of primary care activity interventions, it is recommended that clinicians provide patients with enduring printed material that provides specific information about the exercise program and strategies for addressing barriers (Eakin et al., 2000). As such, we provide in this section links to websites where such material may be obtained. We also include as appendices reproducible handouts that clinicians can provide to patients.

Selecting a form of exercise

In customizing an exercise program, some assessment questions may be helpful to determine factors that may help or hinder a patient's efforts to become more physically active (Meyer & Broocks, 2000; Smith, 2006). First, it is important to assess the patient's experience with and attitudes about exercise. Asking if there have been times when the patient was more physically active than now may help identify activities that were previously enjoyed and the barriers that prevent current participation. It is also valuable to assess the types of exercise resources that are available to the patient. For instance, are there safe locations near the patient's home for walking? Does the patient have access to an exercise facility through their workplace? Does the patient own any exercise equipment in their home such as a treadmill or stationary bicycle? It is also useful to assess the degree of social support patients have in initiating exercise. Are there family members or friends who would be willing to exercise with the patient? Are there co-workers who would be interested in taking walks during a lunch break or before or after work?

In obtaining adherence with a behavioral request, it is important that the assignment be as specific as possible. Thus a patient should not be sent off to begin an exercise program until they have a clear idea of what type and amount of exercise they should do. In deciding on specific types of exercise, the above questions should help to identify types of activities the patient may prefer or have greater ease in accessing. The specific form of exercise is not as important. As noted previously, both aerobic and non-aerobic exercise have been found to be effective in reducing depression, and studies that have directly compared these two types of exercise have not shown a clear advantage for one over the other in terms of symptom reduction (Doyne et al., 1987; Martinsen et al., 1989). Thus patients who are not capable of or motivated to participate in aerobic exercise may expect comparable benefits from non-aerobic exercise such as weightlifting.

Most studies have focused on structured activities taking place either outside of an exercise facility, such as walking, jogging, and running, or activities requiring exercise equipment, such as treadmills, stationary bicycles, and resistance training equipment. However, a variety of daily activities such as housework, yard work, and tasks in some workplaces have the potential to help achieve moderate or vigorous exercise. If such a program of tasks can be routinely implemented, this may be a viable supplement to traditional exercise. A list of such activities and the amount of energy expenditure associated with them can be found on the website for the Centers for Disease Control and Prevention (CDC) (http://www.cdc.gov/nccdphp/dnpa/physical/recommendations/index.htm).

Another low-cost strategy is to encourage patients to purchase a step counter, a device available at most sporting goods stores which quantifies the number of steps taken each day. In a recent forum of leading researchers on exercise and mental health (Otto et al., 2007), it was estimated that depressed individuals may take as few as 2000 to 3000 steps per day compared with the often cited 10,000 steps for a physically active individual. One recommended plan for sedentary individuals is to add 1000 to 2000 steps each week and to work towards the target of 8000 per day.

Self-monitoring forms are often used in research studies to assess adherence with an intervention. However, they can also be useful clinical tools. It may be helpful to ask a patient to record mode of exercise, frequency, and duration on a weekly basis (Trivedi et al., 2006). Such a form may also be useful for recording obstacles to exercise which can then be addressed in follow-up sessions. We provide an example in Appendix A. Furthermore, the mere act of monitoring often influences behavior to change in a desirable direction.

Determining intensity

Another crucial factor in customizing an exercise program is deciding on the target intensity. As reviewed earlier, for reducing depression, it appears that weightlifting is optimally effective at 80% of capacity (Singh et al., 2005). Aerobic exercise is most efficacious at public health recommended dosages of energy expenditure (17.5 kcal/kg/week; Dunn et al., 2005). Individuals who remain at lower dosages tended to show rates of improvement comparable to those in control conditions.

The current public health recommended dosages for physical activity are 30 minutes or more per day of moderate-intensity activities for at least 5 days per week or 20 minutes or more of vigorous intensity activity at least 3 days per week. In helping a patient know at what level of intensity they are completing their activity, there are a number of possible self-monitoring strategies. Again, the CDC website offers reproducible hand-outs on several techniques (http://www.cdc.gov/nccdphp/dnpa/physical/measuring) summarized below. We also summarize several of these in a patient hand-out (Appendix B).

A simple but memorable strategy for monitoring exertion is the talking test. At a light level of activity, a person is typically able to sing. At a moderate level of intensity, a person would be able to carry on a conversation. At a vigorous level of activity, a person is typically too out of breath to have a conversation.

A second strategy is to have patients calculate their target heart rate during the office visit (220 – current age = target heart rate) as well as the range of values associated with physical activity at moderate (50%–70% of target heart rate) and vigorous (70%–85% of target heart rate) levels. During exercise, patients can either monitor their pulse manually or use a portable heart rate device to monitor intensity (Meyer & Broocks, 2000). A third strategy is the use of the Borg's Perceived Level of Exertion Scale (Borg, 1998), a self-report scale with scores ranging from 6 to 20 where patients rate their subjective level of exertion using established anchors. Interestingly, when scores are multiplied by 10, they provide a rough index of actual heart rate. Self-monitoring of heart rate and the Borg's scale have been shown to be feasible in studies with depressed populations (e.g. Armstrong & Edwards, 2004).

As a clinician, it is important to recognize that although optimal dosages have been identified, it may not be initially feasible for all patients. Thus it may be useful to have patients gradually work up to this goal. This graded approach to achieving tasks is consistent with cognitive behavioral therapy (CBT) for at least two reasons. Working up to a treatment target models an incremental approach to problem solving and challenges "all or nothing" thinking common in individuals with depression. If patients simply cannot achieve these recommend target dosages, Stathopoulou et al. (2006) and Singh et al. (2005) note that several studies have shown aerobic exercise to be efficacious at lower dosages. As noted previously, there is some tendency for drop-out to be highest in programs demanding high physical exertion, so there is certainly a risk of non-adherence if a clinician too rigidly demands adherence to a strenuous program.

Once a program has been developed that is satisfactory to both the patient and the clinician, the patient should be encouraged to adhere to the program for at least 4 weeks to help the practice become habit (Meyer & Broocks, 2000). The ultimate goal of self-management is to provide patients with symptom management tools that are enduring beyond the course of treatment by a provider. Therefore, when in doubt, emphasize sustainability over intensity.

Using a trainer

The previous section describes some guidelines and resources for clinicians interested in directly developing an exercise program with a patient. However, as noted previously, this may not be feasible in a number of settings. Therefore, it may be helpful to seek out an exercise professional. It is important to remember that most research studies made some use of trainers who instructed patients in the exercise program and provided ongoing supervision. At a minimum, a trainer may be utilized in a single-session consultation to design an exercise program. For less self-motivated patients, ongoing contact with a trainer may provide additional structure to support maintenance of an exercise program. Trainers can also be helpful in working with patients to prevent exercise-related injuries. In selecting a trainer to refer patients, it is ideal to select professionals certified by national organizations such as the American College of Sports Medicine (ACSM) or the American Council on Exercise (ACE) (Trivedi et al., 2006).

Providing a patient with a long-term exercise supervisor may prove financially and logistically challenging, if not prohibitive. Most insurance plans are unlikely to pay for the services of a trainer. Furthermore, ongoing use of a trainer tends to undermine the goal of using exercise as a self-management strategy. Two recent studies provide examples of how supervised exercise can be transitioned into a self-management program.

In one study, participants engaged in weightlifting supervised for 10 weeks; then participants were asked to continue unsupervised for 10 weeks (Singh et al., 1997). In addition to losing contact with the trainer during this period, participants also had no contact with the researchers. On average, patients completed 18 sessions during the unsupervised period, roughly two workouts a week. As noted previously, nearly a third of all participants were still exercising independently roughly 2 years later.

A recent pilot study by Trivedi et al. (2006) also provides a promising model of integrating self-management and care-management principles to develop a largely self-managed form of treatment with minimal clinician contact. In a 12-week study, participants exercised at the study site for three sessions the first week, two sessions the second week, and one session the third week. During these six sessions, patients worked with a trainer to develop a customized training program. Participants were able to select the type of exercise they preferred, including treadmill, use of a stationary bicycle, above-ground walking, or a combination of these activities. The training program plan included specific details including exercise frequency and appropriate settings for exercise machines. After these 3 weeks, participants transitioned to a fully home-based exercise program, keeping careful logs of home practice. A study staff member remained in telephone contact with participants to troubleshoot adherence issues as needed. Statistical analyses revealed that on average, participants who remained in treatment maintained the exercise programs during the 9 weeks of home practice. In general, mean scores of frequency, duration, and intensity of exercise were constant across the 12 weeks. However, as noted previously, nearly half the participants did not complete the 12-week program.

Both studies highlight how to integrate a professional trainer in a cost-effective manner and provide a combination of structure and flexibility to encourage self-management. Results suggest that a subset of patients is able to make continued use of self-management strategies. However, the majority of patients do not continue these strategies in either the short or long term. This poses a serious challenge to the idea of exercise as a viable self-management strategy.

Recommend a class or group activity

Given the potential financial and logistical challenges of using a trainer, another option for helping to gain the benefits of instruction, structure, and social contact is to refer patients to an exercise class or group activity. As noted previously, it is important to remember that exercise training was conducted in groups; thus social exposure may be a key factor in exercise efficacy. For this reason, it may be helpful to get patients to think about finding a way they can exercise in a group rather than alone.

There are several potential advantages to exercising in a group. First, social isolation and lack of social support have been identified as key factors in maintaining depression. Group exercise has the advantage of forcing the patient to leave his/her home. Given that the demand for deep conversation is low and structure is high in exercise classes or team sports, this may be a less threatening context for patients to re-engage in social situations. Joining a team sport (e.g. community softball league) has the added advantage of providing an experience in which others are counting on the patient to attend regularly, thus making it more difficult to back out on days the patient "doesn't feel like" exercising. Exercise with others can produce additional rewards, such as camaraderie or hearing praise. Such rewards make it more likely that an activity will be repeated. Finally, exercising with others at a similar level of ability can help to keep a person motivated in the face of obstacles and feel a sense of shared struggle with others new to exercise. A person may become more easily frustrated exercising alone or use unrealistic standards of comparison (e.g. the most physically fit person at the gym).

Make the first step easier

Depressed patients participating in a pilot study of an exercise intervention revealed that a large obstacle to initiating exercise is making the initial contact with a fitness center (Seime & Vickers, 2006). Patients in this study were grateful that the study staff had assisted them in setting up the initial appointment and could answer questions about the fitness center. It may be useful for a clinician to educate him or herself about a range of fitness centers in the areas of varying cost (e.g. private fitness clubs, community centers, hospital-based gyms, YMCAs) and what is required for obtaining a membership and a consultation with an exercise professional. As noted in the section on roles, it may be helpful to develop a list of exercise professionals to whom the clinician may refer the client. Finally, it may be helpful to take the first step for the patient in setting up the initial appointment at a fitness center if the patient agrees to waive the necessary confidentiality protections. This could be accomplished by a clinician during the treatment visit or by clinical support staff afterwards.

Enhancing motivation

In the previous section, we discussed various external supporting factors that can be employed, including the treating clinicians, trainers, and other exercisers. In this section, we discuss strategies for cultivating the patient's internal motivation to exercise.

Tailor the message

As noted previously, gaining compliance with an exercise regimen may be especially difficult due to the effects of depression on motivation and energy levels. Thus it is crucial that a patient have some belief that the treatment will be effective for him or her. Like with pharmacotherapy or psychotherapy, it is valuable that the clinicians explain to the patient why he or she believes the treatment will help. It is important to match a treatment rationale to the patient's own model of understanding his/her disorder. The earlier section on proposed mechanisms in this chapter can be a valuable resource for the clinician in this regard. For a patient who understands his/her symptoms primarily from a somatic perspective, it may be valuable to highlight some of the proposed biological mechanisms. For the patient who takes a more interpersonal approach, the social benefits of joining a group exercise may be more persuasive. For the patient who emphasizes self-esteem or tends to ruminate on personal inadequacies, a clinician may wish to emphasize the potential for exercise to enhance self-esteem or to provide an active distraction from ruminative thinking. We include a list of these mechanisms along with a brief summary of intervention research in a patient hand-out included at the end of this chapter (Appendix C).

Help the patient find his or her own motivation

One of the biggest challenges in helping an individual with depression to exercise can be the perceived lack of motivation to initiate new activities. Motivational interviewing (Miller & Rollnick, 1991) is a technique that was developed initially for the treatment of substance abuse and dependence but has been subsequently applied to other health promotion behaviors. Similar strategies can be applied in helping the patient with depression find their motivation to begin exercising. One technique would be to help the patient first think about the pros and cons of exercising. We included a patient hand-out that may be helpful in presenting this activity to a patient (Appendix D). Next, ask the patient to list the pros and cons of remaining sedentary. If asking for "pros and cons" seems to produce more intellectualized answers rather than answers that seem personally salient for the patient, consider asking them to think about times when they were more physically active and what they liked about it. What was hard in maintaining it? What do you like about being less active currently? Is there anything that troubles you about your current habits?

By asking patients to develop their own reasons, the clinician will find what resonates with particular patients and can help them discover their own motivations to change. A large principle of motivational interviewing (MI) is the use of active listening while refraining from persuasion, asserting expertise, argument, or other more active tactics to change the patient's mind. However, it may be helpful to gently guide a patient in critically evaluating his/her lists of "pros of remaining sedentary" and "cons of becoming more active" to see if there aren't other more helpful ways of viewing these barriers to change or strategies that can be used to cope with these obstacles.

This list may also become a valuable resource if the patient's motivation wanes. Patients might be encouraged to keep a copy of this list with them in a place where it would be easy to access it when they are tempted to skip exercise (e.g. bedside table, in the car, on top of the television set).

Anticipate obstacles and strategies

As noted previously, problem solving may be especially challenging for patients with depression. For this reason, it may be helpful to try to anticipate obstacles with the patient in advance to prevent some barriers and maximize the likelihood of early success. For instance, an individual who reports being too busy to find time to exercise could be coached on time management, how to make exercise a priority, or how to make daily activities more physically strenuous. An individual who reports being too tired to exercise at the end of the day could be coached to try working out in the morning or to break their workout into shorter 10-minute increments throughout the day. A helpful brochure is available from the National Institute of Health and US Department of Health and Human Services (http://win.niddk.nih.gov/publications/PDFs/tipsactive.pdf) which contains a list of common barriers and simple strategies for addressing them. Patients may be referred to this as a self-management tool or a practitioner may use it as a reference when troubleshooting with a patient.

Maintaining the practice and commitment

As noted previously, adherence to exercise can be a challenge for individuals with depression. For this reason, it is important that a clinician use strategies to help maintain a patient's commitment. This can include providing ongoing support, encouragement, and reinforcement of all efforts made. Follow-up phone calls may help to raise levels of adherence (Craft & Perna, 2004). Patients with depression may respond to initial lapses such as missing exercise sessions with frustration, self-criticism, and hopelessness about the likelihood of future successes; thus it may be important to point out that such patterns of thinking will undermine continued efforts (Seime & Vickers, 2006).

As noted previously, some anticipatory troubleshooting may help to prevent some initial barriers. However, it is likely that new barriers will present themselves once participants engage with the exercise. Below are some possible obstacles and strategies for addressing them.

Some patients might find the selected activity to be tedious, in which case it might be possible to recommend that the patient listen to music or an audiobook during exercise. In fact, downloading or purchasing new music or audiobooks after a certain number of completed exercise sessions may be useful as a self-administered reward. Alternatively, inviting a friend for company or walking in a stimulating environment such as a park or shopping mall may help make exercise more pleasurable.

Some may find exercise aversive in that it becomes a relatively distraction-free time in which ruminative thoughts become overwhelming. In these instances, it may be helpful to coach the patient in the use of techniques from mindfulness meditation during exercise. In one study, patients were instructed to respond to ruminative thinking by turning attention to their own breathing, the sound and feeling of their feet as they made contact with the running surface, and the sensation of having their spine being erect as they ran (Greist et al., 1979).

Some patients will report not having sufficient energy to exercise. As noted previously, it can be helpful to examine times of the day when they are more likely to have energy or to break down exercising into smaller units. It may also help to remind patients to drink sufficient quantities of water when exercising to prevent feelings of fatigue resulting from dehydration. Patients may need to be reminded that exercise will help create energy and feelings of vitality, but requires an initial investment of energy. In fact, one study demonstrated that a single 30-minute exercise session was able to produce increased positive affect and vigor in patients with depression (Bartholomew et al., 2005).

If the patient has not started exercising or is perilously close to quitting, it may be helpful to revisit the list of pros and cons generated earlier in treatment. It is possible that reviewing the advantages of exercise and the downsides of remaining sedentary may provide encouragement to continue coping with barriers. This may also be a point in which modification of goals is useful. If this is done, care should be taken to present this modification as an example of effective problem solving instead of an indication that the patient has "failed."

Summary and conclusions

This chapter has reviewed the body of literature on exercise as a treatment for depression. Studies have shown that exercise can be effective at reducing symptoms of depression and is consistent with the goals of self-management. However, there is considerable evidence that adherence to exercise tends to reduce outside of supervised exercise settings. This may be due to the demanding nature of exercise as well as the symptoms and psychopathology of depression. The final portion of the chapter presented recommendations for optimizing the likelihood that patients will adhere to an exercise program by providing appropriate supports and working to enhance patients' own motivation and helping them to overcome barriers to exercise.

REFERENCES

Armstrong K, Edwards H. The effectiveness of a pram-walking exercise programme in reducing depressive symptomatology for postnatal women. *Int J Nurs Pract.* 2004; 10(4):177–194.

Babyak M, Blumenthal J, Herman S, Khatri P, Doraiswamy M, Moore K, Craighead WE, Baldewicz TT, Krishnan KR. Exercise treatment for major depression: maintenance of therapeutic benefit at 10 months. *Psychosom Med.* 2000; 62(5):633–638.

Bartholomew JB, Morrison D, Ciccolo JT. Effects of acute exercise on mood and well-being in patients with major depressive disorder. *Med Sci Sports Exerc.* 2005; 37(12):2032–2037.

Biddle SJH. Emotion, mood, and physical activity. In Biddle SJH, Fox KR, and Boutcher SH, eds: *Physical Activity and Psychological Well-Being.* London: Routledge; 2000.

Blumenthal JA, Babyak MA, Moore KA, Craighead WE, Herman S, Khatri P, Waugh R, Napolitano MA, Forman LM, Appelbaum M, Doraiswamy PM, Krishnan KR. Effects of exercise training on older patients with major depression. *Arch Intern Med.* 1999; 159:2349–2356.

Borg G. *Borg's Perceived Exertion and Pain Scales.* Champaign, IL: Human Kinetics; 1998.

Bosscher R. Running and mixed physical exercises with depressed psychiatric patients. *Int J Sport Psychol.* 1993; 24(2):170–184.

Chambless D, Hollon S. Defining empirically supported therapies. *J Consult Clin Psychol.* 1998; 66(1):7–18.

Craft LL. Exercise and clinical depression: examining two psychological mechanisms. *Psychol Sport Exerc.* 2005; 6:151–171.

Craft LL, Perna FM. The benefits of exercise for the clinically depressed. *Prim Care Companion J Clin Psychiatry.* 2004; 6(3):104–113.

Dimidjian S, Hollon S, Dobson KS, Schmaling KB, Kohlenberg RJ, Addis ME, Gallop R, McGlinchey JB, Markley DK, Gollan JK, Atkins DC, Dunner DL, Jacobson NS. Randomized trial of behavioral activation, cognitive therapy, and antidepressant medication in the acute treatment of adults with major depression. *J Consult Clin Psychol.* 2006; 74:658–670

Dishman RK. Mental health. In Seefeldt V, ed: *Mental Health.* Reston, VA: American Alliance for Health, Physical Education, Recreation and Dance; 1986, pp 303–341.

Doyne EJ, Ossip-Klein DJ, Bowman ED, Osborn KM, McDougall-Wilson IB, Neimeyer RA. Running versus weight lifting in the treatment of depression. *J Consult Clin Psychol.* 1987; 55(5):748–754.

Dunn A, Trivedi M, Kampert J, Clark C, Chambliss H. Exercise treatment for depression: efficacy and dose response. *Am J Prev Med.* 2005; 28(1):1–8.

Eakin EG, Glasgow RE, Riley KM. Review of primary care-based physical activity intervention studies: effectiveness and implications for practice and future research. *J Fam Pract.* 2000; 49:158–68.

Ernst C, Olson AK, Pinel JPJ, Lam RW, Christie BR. Antidepressant effects of exercise: evidence for an adult-neurogenesis hypothesis? *J Psychiatry Neurosci.* 2006; 31(2):84–92.

Feldman GC. Cognitive and behavioral therapies for depression: overview, new directions, and practical recommendations for dissemination. *Psychiatr Clin North Am.* 2007; 30(1):39–50.

Fremont J, Craighead LW. Aerobic exercise and cognitive therapy in the treatment of dysphoric moods. *Cognit Ther Res.* 1987; 11(2):241–251.

Greist JH, Klein MH, Eischens RR, Faris J, Gurman AS, Morgan WP. Running as treatment for depression. *Compr Psychiatry.* 1979; 20(1):41–54.

Herman S, Blumenthal JA, Babyak M, Khatri P, Craighead WE, Krishnan KR, Doraiswamy PM. Exercise therapy for depression in middle-aged and older adults: predictors of early dropout and treatment failure. *Health Psychol.* 2002; 21(6):553–563.

Hopko D, Lejuez C, Ruggiero K, Eifert G. Contemporary behavioral activation treatments for depression: procedures, principles and progress. *Clin Psychol Rev.* 2003; 23(5):699–717.

Hughes JR. Psychological effects of habitual aerobic exercise: a critical review. *Prev Med.* 1984; 13(1):66–67.

Klein MH, Greist JH, Gurman AS, Neimeyer RA, Lesser DP, Bushnell NJ, et al. A comparative outcome study of group psychotherapy vs. exercise treatments for depression. *Int J Ment Health.* 1985; 16(3–4):148–177.

Kubesch S, Bretschneider V, Freudenmann R, Weidenhammer N, Lehmann M, Spitzer M, Grön G. Aerobic endurance exercise improves executive functions in depressed patients. *J Clin Psychiatry.* 2003; 64(9):1005–1012.

Larun L, Nordheim LV, Ekeland E, Hagen KB, Heian F. Exercise in prevention and treatment of anxiety and depression among children and young people. *Cochrane Database Syst Rev.* 2006; 3:CD004691.

Lawlor D, Hopker S. The effectiveness of exercise as an intervention in the management of depression: systematic review and meta-regression analysis of randomised controlled trials. *BMJ.* 2001; 322(7289):763–766.

Martinsen EW. Benefits of exercise for the treatment of depression. *Sports Med.* 1990; 9(6):380–389.

Martinsen EW, Hoffart A, Solberg O. Comparing aerobic with nonaerobic forms of exercise in the treatment of clinical depression: a randomized trial. *Compr Psychiatry.* 1989; 30:234–331.

Martinsen EW, Medhus A, Sandvik L. Effects of aerobic exercise on depression: a controlled study. *BMJ.* 1985; 291:109.

Mather A, Rodriguez C, Guthrie M, McHarg A, Reid I, McMurdo M. Effects of exercise on depressive symptoms in older adults with poorly responsive depressive disorder: randomised controlled trial. *Br J Psychiatry.* 2002; 180(5):411–415.

McNeil J, LeBlanc E, Joyner M. The effect of exercise on depressive symptoms in the moderately depressed elderly. *Psychol Aging.* 1991; 6(3):487–488.

Meyer T, Broocks A. Therapeutic impact of exercise on psychiatric diseases: guidelines for exercise testing and prescription. *Sports Med.* 2000; 30:269–279.

Miller W, Rollnick S. *Motivational Interviewing: Preparing People to Change Addictive Behavior.* New York, NY: Guilford Press; 1991.

Morgan WP. Selected physiological and psychomotor correlates of depression in psychiatric patients. *Res Q.* 1968; 39:1037–1043.

Otto MW, Church TS, Craft LL, Greer TL, Smits JAJ, Trivedi MH. Exercise for mood and anxiety disorders. *J Clin Psychiatry.* 2007; 9(4):287–294.

Rush AJ, Trivedi MH, Wisniewski SR, Nierenberg AA, Stewart JW, Warden D, Niederehe G, Thase ME, Lavori PW, Lebowitz BD, McGrath PJ, Rosenbaum JF, Sackeim HA, Kupfer DJ, Luther J, Fava M. Acute and longer-term outcomes in depressed outpatients requiring one or several treatment steps: A STAR*D report. *Am J Psychiatry.* 2006; 163(11):1905–1917.

Seime R, Vickers K. The challenges of treating depression with exercise: from evidence to practice. *Clin Psychol Sci Pract.* 2006; 13(2):194–197.

Sexton H, Mære Å, Dahl N. Exercise intensity and reduction in neurotic symptoms: a controlled follow-up study. *Acta Psychiatr Scand.* 1989; 80(3):231–235.

Singh N. A randomized controlled trial of high versus low intensity weight training versus general practitioner care for clinical depression in older adults. *J Gerontol A Biol Sci Med Sci.* 2005; 60A:768–776.

Singh N, Clements K, Fiatarone M. A randomized controlled trial of progressive resistance training in depressed elders. *J Gerontol A Biol Sci Med Sci.* 1997; 52(1): M27–M35.

Singh N, Clements K, Fiatarone Singh M. The efficacy of exercise as a long-term antidepressant in elderly subjects: a randomized, controlled trial. *J Gerontol A Biol Sci Med Sci.* 2001; 56(8):M497–M504.

Singh N, Stavrinos T, Scarbek Y, Galambos G, Liber C, Singh F. A randomized controlled trial of high versus low intensity weight training versus general practitioner care for clinical depression in older adults. *J Gerontol A Biol Sci Med Sci.* 2005; 60A:768–776.

Sjösten N, Kivelä S. The effects of physical exercise on depressive symptoms among the aged: a systematic review. *Int J Geriatr Psychiatry.* 2006; 21(5):410–418.

Smith T. Blood, sweat, and tears: exercise in the management of mental and physical health problems. *Clin Psychol Sci Pract.* 2006; 13(2):198–202.

Stathopoulou G, Powers M, Berry A, Smits J, Otto M. Exercise interventions for mental health: a quantitative and qualitative review. *Clin Psychol Sci Pract.* 2006; 13(2):179–193.

Trivedi M, Greer T, Grannemann B, Chambliss H, Jordan A. Exercise as an augmentation strategy for treatment of major depression. *J Psychiatr Pract.* 2006; 12(4):205–211.

Van Der Pompe G, Bernards N, Meijman T, Heijnen C. The effect of depressive symptomatology on plasma cortisol responses to acute bicycle exercise among postmenopausal women. *Psychiatry Res.* 1999; 85(1):113–117.

Veale D, Le Fevre K, Pantelis C, de Souza V, Mann A, Sargeant A. Aerobic exercise in the adjunctive treatment of depression: a randomized controlled trial. *J R Soc Med.* 1992; 85:541–544.

Appendix A   Weekly exercise log

For each time you exercise this week, please record the date, activity, time, and duration. If you exercise more than once in the same day, please use a separate line to record this.

Date	Activity	Time-spent exercising (in minutes)	Heart rate during exercise (beats per minute)	Distance in miles (if walking, running or biking)

Please describe any obstacles you encountered this week that made it difficult to meet your exercise goals:

Source: Based upon materials developed by presented by Madhukar Trivedi, M.D. and colleagues (see Trivedi M, Greer T, Grannemann B, Chambliss H, Jordan A. Exercise as an augmentation strategy for treatment of major depression. *J Psychiatr Pract.* 2006; 12(4):205–211).

APPENDIX B   Tips for deciding on type, schedule, and intensity of exercise

What type of exercise is right for me?

Most studies have focused on structured activities taking place either outside of an exercise facility, such as walking, jogging, and running, or activities requiring exercise equipment, such as treadmills, stationary bicycles, and resistance training equipment. However, a variety of daily activates such as housework, yard work, and tasks in some workplaces have the potential to help achieve moderate or vigorous activity. A list of such activities and the amount of energy expenditure associated with them can be found on the website for the Centers for Disease Control and Prevention (CDC) (http://www.cdc.gov/nccdphp/dnpa/physical/recommendations/index.htm).

There are a few other factors it may be helpful to consider. First, consider an activity that you have enjoyed in the past. It might be easier to resume something familiar than trying something entirely new. Second, it is also worth considering structuring your exercise so you are not doing it alone. When you exercise with a partner, you can help keep each other motivated. Similarly, joining an exercise class or a team sport in the community can help provide support and rewarding social interactions as you develop your new healthy habit.

How much exercise should I be doing to help manage depression?

This question is less straightforward than it may appear. One way to answer it is that even a small amount of exercise is always better than no exercise. Whatever amount you decide upon, remember two rules of thumb:

- It is more realistic to start with a small amount of exercise and work up to larger amounts gradually. This will allow your body to get used to being active and help make your first efforts at exercise more pleasant.
- It is better to develop a routine that helps you exercise in small doses on a regular schedule rather than doing the occasional, irregular burst of a lot of exercise. This plan is more sustainable in the long term and more likely to become habit. It is important that you stick with your activity for at least 4 weeks to help the practice become habit.

How intense should my exercise be?

Researchers have only recently begun to study the optimal "dose" of exercise to treat depression. The current public health recommended dosages for physical activity are 30 minutes or more per day of moderate-intensity activities for at least 5 days per week or 20 minutes or more of vigorous intensity activity at least 3 days per week. This amount also seems to be helpful for depression as well. However, if you have not been physically active for a while, it is wise to work up to this amount over the course of a few weeks.

How do I know if my exercise is moderate or vigorous?

There are several methods for determining the intensity of your exercise.

Method 1: What activity are you doing?
The Centers for Disease Control and Prevention published on their website a list of different types of exercise and daily activity that fall into each of these categories (http://www.cdc.gov/nccdphp/dnpa/physical/recommendations/index.htm).

For instance, riding a bike 5 to 9 miles an hour on level ground would be moderate; more than 10 miles an hour or riding up a steep hill would be more vigorous. Shooting baskets is moderate; playing basketball is vigorous. This list may also be helpful for giving you ideas about activities to add to your daily routine to increase your activity level.

Method 2: The talking test

A simple but memorable strategy for monitoring exertion is the talking test. At a light level of activity, a person is typically able to sing. At a moderate level of intensity, a person would be able to carry on a conversation. At a vigorous level of activity, a person is typically too out of breath to have a conversation. Obviously, this test works best if you are exercising with someone you know. However, if you are exercising alone, no one will know if you are singing or talking aloud to yourself!

Method 3: How fast is your heart beating?

Another method involves keeping track of how fast your heart is beating during exercise. In a moment, we will explain how to do this. However, first it is important to determine your target heart rate and the heart rates that are associated with moderate and vigorous activity levels:

Step 1: Subtract your current age from 220.

220	$-$	_____	$=$	_____
		Current age		Target heart beat

Step 2: Use the formulas below to calculate the range of heart rate scores associated with moderate and vigorous levels of activity.

Moderate activity level (50%–70% of Target Heart Rate):

_____	$\times$	.50	$=$	_____
Target Heart Beat				Low end of moderate (50%)
_____	$\times$	.70	$=$	_____
Target Heart Beat				High end of moderate (70%)

Vigorous activity level (70%–85% of Target Heart Rate):

_____	$\times$	.70	$=$	_____
Target Heart Beat				Low end of vigorous (75%)
_____	$\times$	.85	$=$	_____
Target Heart Beat				High end of vigorous (85%)

Once you know your target numbers, you can monitor your heart rate one of two ways. The easiest is to use a portable device to monitor your heart rate available at most sporting goods stores. An equally effective "low-tech" method involves the following steps:

1. Stop exercising for a moment.
2. Press the tips of your index and middle finger of your right hand on the wrist of your left arm. Your finger tips should be directly below the palm of your left hand, in line with the index finger of your left hand. You should be able to feel your pulse.
3. Once you feel your pulse, begin timing 60 seconds on your watch and count the number of pulses you feel during that time. Alternatively, you can count for 30 seconds and then double the number. To obtain the most accurate number, start timing on the first pulse, which should be counted as "zero."

Source: Centers for Disease Control and Prevention (CDC)

APPENDIX C   Frequently asked questions about exercise and depression treatment

Does exercise help to reduce depression symptoms?

Yes. According to many studies, people with depression who were assigned to begin an exercise program show much greater improvement in their symptoms compared with people who were placed on a waiting list or asked to participate in an alternative activity, such as attending lectures on health. A few studies have suggested that people who begin a structured exercise program may show improvements in depression symptoms that are similar to those of people receiving antidepressant medication or structured counseling. It is also possible that exercise might be a helpful next step for people who have already begun medication but have not fully recovered.

What kind of exercise is most helpful?

Studies have shown benefits for both aerobic exercise, like walking, jogging, and riding a stationary bike, as well as non-aerobic exercise, like weightlifting. It is important that each person choose a form and schedule of exercise that is the right match for them based on their lifestyle and current physical condition. Your health care provider can help you set realistic goals to increase your likelihood of success.

Why does exercise reduce depression?

There is no one definitive answer to this question. It is likely that exercise produces many benefits simultaneously, and it may produce different benefits for different people. Researchers are continuing to learn more about the benefits of exercise for mental health. The following is a list of reasons drawn from existing research which suggests how exercise can help reduce depression:

- *Brain benefits*: Exercise may help promote the growth of brain cells and regulate brain chemicals called neurotransmitters in a manner similar to other medical treatments for depression. Exercise may also help to activate the prefrontal cortex, an area of the brain that is involved in concentrating and making decisions.
- *Body benefits*: Exercise may also help to normalize levels of stress hormones in the body. By increasing energy levels and normalizing sleep, exercise may also work directly on two key physical symptoms of depression.
- *Psychological benefits*: Successfully beginning an exercise program may increase feelings of competence and self-esteem. The habit of regular exercise can help break less healthy habits associated with depression, including withdrawing from people and life in general. Exercise can also provide a healthy distraction from self-critical thoughts and dwelling on how badly one feels, a process called depressive rumination.

Brain, body, and psychological benefits can work together. For instance, if exercise works to increase concentration, energy, and confidence, it may become easier for people to stick with their efforts to accomplish important goals or tackle lingering problems.

How do I get started?

Now that you know a bit more about the science behind exercise as a treatment for depression, you may be more willing to give it a try as a strategy for managing your symptoms. If so, talk to your health care provider about ways to get started!

Source: For more information on the research findings described above, you may wish to read *Self-Management of Depression* by Albert Yeung, M.D., Sc.D.; Greg Feldman, Ph.D.; & Maurizio Fava, M.D. Cambridge University Press.

APPENDIX D   The pros and cons of beginning to exercise

Changing any habit can be tough. One reason for this is that people typically have mixed feelings about making a change. For that reason, it can be helpful to review the pros and cons of both changing and staying the same to gain a full picture of the different thoughts and feelings you have about changing. Please use the table on the following page to write down the benefits and costs of exercising and not exercising *as you see them*. Try to answer these questions in a way that is true for you, not what you think you are "supposed" to write or how other people would answer them. There are no right and wrong answers.

	Benefits / Pros *Q. What do you like about getting more exercise? (Example: "Having more energy")*	**Cost / Cons** *Q. What concerns you about getting more exercise? (Example: "Might feel embarrassed exercising around people")*
Making a change (Exercising more)		
	Q. What do you like about your current activity level? (Example: "Most of my hobbies are low-key: watching TV, hanging out with friends . . .")	*Q. What concerns you about your current activity level? (Example: "Don't like getting winded when walking up stairs")*
Not changing (Maintaining current activity level)		

Once you have completed this exercise, discuss it with your health care provider. On a separate sheet of paper, please write out all of the reasons you listed in the two grey boxes. If you decide to begin exercising, keep a copy of this list in a place where it will be easy to review it at moments when you are trying to decide if you will exercise, for example, your bedside table, in your car, on top of your television set. Keeping this list handy can help you stick with your exercise goals in the face of temptation to be sedentary.

Source: Based on an exercise developed by William R. Miller, Ph.D., and Stephen Rollnick, Ph.D. (See Miller W, Rollnick S. *Motivational Interviewing: Preparing People to Change Addictive Behavior.* New York: Guilford Press; 1991).

Self-management of depression using meditation

There are various forms of meditation that have been practiced across different cultures for centuries. The word meditation comes from the Latin *meditatio*, which originally indicated every type of physical or intellectual exercise, but later evolved into the more specific meaning of "contemplation." In the West, meditation is viewed as a strategy of self-regulation, with a particular focus on training one's attention. On the other hand, in the East, meditation is usually practiced to cultivate calmness, concentration, and positive emotions (Goleman, 1988). Walsh and Shapiro (2006) attempted to integrate the two different views and defined meditation as "a family of self-regulation practices that focuses on training attention and awareness in order to bring mental processes under greater voluntary control and thereby foster general mental well-being and development and/or specific capacities such as calm, clarity, and concentration." In the past several decades, considerable evidence has emerged that meditation may be an effective form of stress management and thus be useful in the treatment of a variety of medical and psychiatric conditions, including depression.

In this chapter, we will first discuss how meditation is relevant as a self-management tool. We will then talk about some of the more widely researched and practiced forms of meditation. Next we will discuss how meditation may address both biological and cognitive factors that are relevant to the disease process of depression. We will then review the clinical research literature, which demonstrates how various forms of meditation may help reduce depression and anxiety symptoms across a variety of populations. The literature consists of studies that examine meditation as a treatment for clinical depression and some that specifically look at meditation as a form of relapse prevention. Following this review, we will discuss the current state of the field and what remains to be learned about the efficacy of meditation in the management of depression. Finally, we will conclude with a discussion of practical issues that clinicians should consider upon recommending meditation as a treatment plan for depression.

Why is meditation useful for self-management of depression?

Meditation has considerable potential as a form of self-management. Once learned, meditation techniques can be self-administered to regulate levels of arousal and tension. It can also become an alternative activity that one may use to help disrupt the repetitive cycles of depressive rumination. One goal of self-management interventions is to help individuals manage prodromal depression symptoms in order to prevent relapse into full episodes. In particular, it may be helpful for individuals who are at risk for future episodes of depression to learn to increase awareness of their thoughts, emotions, and somatic symptoms, any of which may signal a return of depression, and to respond to these signals with adaptive emotion regulation strategies. Meditation may be one such approach. As we will review in detail, two recent studies suggest that mindfulness meditation can help to prevent relapse in individuals with chronic, recurrent depression (three or more previous episodes). As we discussed in Chapter 1, individuals with chronic forms of depression may be those who would benefit most from such self-management. Consistent with other self-management strategies, meditation may require some initial instruction and follow-up from a clinician to help support the cultivation of this new habit. However, once sufficient support has been provided for the development of these skills, meditation has considerable promise to become an effective form of self-management, with potential benefits for a wide range of health issues and with little or no side effects.

What is meditation?

Practiced for over five millennia, meditation is recognized as a component of almost all world religions. Meditative practices are found in traditions in both Eastern and Western cultures, including Christianity, Islam, and Judaism. The most popular forms of meditation in the Western world over the last half century are the Buddhist and Indian forms, including various Yoga forms (Arias et al., 2006). In recent times, Western culture has increasingly adopted and practiced Eastern meditation techniques, and researchers and clinicians have introduced secular versions of meditation as well, under the names of relaxation response training (Benson, 1975) and mindfulness meditation (Kabat-Zinn, 1990). In the past three decades, mind–body techniques, which include meditation, yoga, and Tai Chi, among others, have gained increasing popularity in the United States. In showing the importance of meditation as a therapeutic tool, Walsh and Shapiro (2006) pointed out that, with an estimated 10 million practitioners in the United States, meditation is now one of the world's most enduring and widely practiced and researched psychological disciplines.

Numerous forms of meditation exist, and they are usually classified according to their focus. Many meditative practices simply focus one's attention on the breath. In fact, this is a natural object of meditation as the mind can become absorbed into the rhythm of inhalation and exhalation. Frequently, during meditation, one's breathing rhythm slows and deepens, leading the mind to become quiet and more aware. Some meditative practices simply attend to, without judgment, one's thoughts, emotions, sensations, and perceptions as they arise moment by moment in one's field of awareness; this is called "mindfulness meditation" (Astin et al., 2003). Other meditative practices focus on a preselected specific object; this is called "concentration meditation" (Barrows & Jacobs, 2002). In practice, many forms of meditative techniques meld mindfulness and concentration meditations.

To practice mindfulness meditation, the meditator sits silently and tries to simply become aware of the continuous flow of sensations, feelings, images, thoughts, sounds, smells, and whatever else the mind experiences, while paying attention to their breathing. The goal is to not think about or become involved with the thoughts, memories, worries, or images that may spring up. By quietly detaching the mind in this way, mindfulness meditation allows the mind to become calmer, clearer, and more non-reactive, a state that lets the body's own inner wisdom be heard. If during mindfulness meditation, the practitioners notice their attention wandering, they are supposed to simply observe the process without trying to disengage from it and to return to awareness of their breathing. Ultimately, to practice mindfulness meditation, the practitioner, with a "no effort" attitude, is encouraged to maintain an open focus where one perception shifts freely into the next: no thought, image, or sensation is considered an intrusion, but simply an awareness of being in the here and now.

Whereas in mindfulness meditation there is an open focus, in concentration meditation, the practitioners fix their attention on a particular object. Concentration meditation is usually done in a quiet place, where the practitioner, once seated in a comfortable position, adopts a passive attitude and starts to meditate with a repetitive mental stimulus. People who practice concentration meditation often choose an image, a word, a sound, or a short phrase as their mental stimulus. They would then return to this image or repeat this word/sound/phrase with each in-breath while sitting in a relaxed position with their eyes closed. Should any distracting thoughts and feelings arise while meditating, the practitioners would simply dismiss such distractions calmly and return their attention to their chosen mental stimulus. By focusing on the image, word, or sound, distractions are minimized and the mind is quieted to achieve a greater awareness and clarity. Concentration meditation is often used in religious and spiritual practices.

While many forms of meditations are practiced in a seated position, there are also other forms of meditation practices. Meditation can also be practiced while walking or doing simple repetitive tasks. Walking meditation helps to focus attention on the process of becoming aware of oneself while moving in a physically familiar manner. Additional examples of meditative practices involving movement include various types of yoga, which has received increasing acceptance in the West in the past decades. Yoga originated from Indian philosophy and religion, but the practice of yoga does not require spiritual beliefs or religious observances. Practice of yoga involves multiple dimensions: the learning of essential ethical principles for living; physical postures for development of strength, flexibility, and endurance; breathing practices for promoting concentration; and meditation for promoting awareness. Based on these principles, different yogic disciplines have been developed, including Raja, Mantra, Jnana, Karma, and Bhakti yoga. The most common aspects of yoga practiced in the West are the physical postures and breathing practices of Hatha yoga (an aspect of Raja yoga) and meditation (Collins, 1998). Regardless of whether one is sitting still or moving about, ultimately the goal of meditation is to bring about greater personal awareness. Although meditation has been practiced for centuries, its benefits in terms of mental and physical health have only begun to receive systematic study in the past five decades. In particular, three meditation programs have received the greatest scientific study: Transcendental Meditation, the Relaxation Response, and Mindfulness-Based Stress Reduction. We describe each of these approaches briefly below and later discuss the research supporting these as well as other forms of meditation in basic and clinical studies.

Transcendental Meditation (TM) was introduced by Maharishi Mahesh Yogi in the late 1950s and is described in his book *The Science of Being and Art of Living: Transcendental Meditation* (1963) as a form of concentration meditation, which is based upon techniques derived from the Vedas, the oldest sacred texts of Hinduism. This technique gained worldwide attention when Western celebrities including members of the Beatles traveled to India to study TM with him in the late 1960s. TM is practiced twice daily for 15 to 20 minutes. Individuals practicing TM are taught to sit comfortably with their eyes closed for two 15- to 20-minute sessions per day and to focus their attention on a mantra, a word that is silently repeated. Instruction in TM is typically provided by teachers who have undergone a specific training program.

In addition to TM, two other meditation programs have been introduced to Western health care settings by two pioneering researchers. Herbert Benson introduced a comprehensive program, popularized in his book *The Relaxation Response* (1975). He developed a variation of Transcendental Meditation (TM), which was easier to learn than the original, but could still elicit a series of positive mental and physical changes. Benson noted that having a mental device on which to focus one's attention, a passive attitude toward distracting thoughts, a comfortable position to allow decreased muscle tone, and a quiet environment were the four important elements to produce this response, which he named the Relaxation Response (RR). Although this program includes many forms of relaxation techniques, perhaps the most well-known approach is a form of concentrative meditation in which meditators count individual breaths and focus on a single word. Unlike TM, where a special mantra is chosen by the instructor, the individual practicing Benson's technique can select a word or short phrase, such as "peace" or "calm," which is meaningful to them.

Jon Kabat-Zinn, the second research pioneer in this field, is credited with introducing mindfulness meditation to a broad audience and conducting some of the first studies of this approach. Mindfulness is defined as the awareness of one's thoughts, actions, or motivations. Mindfulness plays a central role in Buddhist teachings, where it is affirmed that "correct" or "right" mindfulness is an essential factor in the path to liberation from *samsara*, the cycle of death and rebirth and all the suffering and limitations of worldly existence. Such mindfulness helps meditators use their inner resources to achieve good health and well-being. Kabat-Zinn introduced an 8-week stress management course, named Mindfulness-Based Stress Reduction program (MBSR), which combines meditation and Hatha yoga to help patients cope with stress, pain, and illness by using moment-to-moment awareness. The program is described in his book *Full Catastrophe Living* (Kabat-Zinn, 1990). Of particular relevance to this chapter, MBSR has been adapted into an intervention to prevent relapse of depression in recovered patients. This intervention has been named Mindfulness-Based Cognitive Therapy (MBCT; Segal et al., 2002) and, as we discuss in a later section, is currently being tested as a treatment for depression.

What are the possible mechanisms for meditation to reduce depression?

Traditionally, people used metaphors like "purifying the mind," "rebalancing the mental elements," "awakening the mind from its usual trance," or, for those with a more religious outlook, "enlightening/uncovering true identity" to explain how contemplation works (Walsh & Shapiro, 2006). Many of these metaphors reflect how the brain was viewed: as an organic machine that undergoes a developmental process. Contemporary explanations of the mechanisms of meditation embody the integration of both mind and body and recognize their interplay. In this section, we discuss two possible mechanisms of meditation that are especially relevant for depression: (1) alleviation of the effect of stress on the hypothalamic-pituitary-adrenal axis, and (2) cognitive changes, including enhanced regulation of attention and de-identification with negative thoughts.

Meditation may alleviate the effect of stress on the hypothalamic-pituitary-adrenal axis

There are various possible biological mechanisms by which meditation can help reduce the symptoms of depression. One possible mechanism is through the hypothalamic-pituitary-adrenal (HPA) axis, a major part of the neuroendocrine system that manages reactions to stress and regulates various processes in the body, including digestion, energy usage, the immune system, and mood. The HPA axis is a complex set of direct influences and homeostatic feedback interactions between the hypothalamus, which is responsible for certain metabolic processes and various activities of the autonomic nervous system; the pituitary gland, which secretes hormones regulating homeostasis; and the adrenal glands, which are responsible for regulating the stress response through the synthesis of corticosteroids and catecholamines, including cortisol and adrenaline. Species from humans to the most ancient organisms share components of the HPA axis, which helps mediate adaptation with its various interactions. Since it plays such a large role in the neuroendocrine system, the HPA axis has been hypothesized to be involved in the neurobiology of clinical depression, panic symptoms, and post-traumatic stress disorder (Swaab et al., 2005; Yehuda et al., 1991; Abelson et al., 2007).

The relationship between the hypothalamic-pituitary-adrenal axis and depression

Although the exact mechanism of clinical depression is still unclear, evidence has suggested that stress probably plays an important role in this disorder, perhaps through its effects on the HPA axis (Pariante, 2003). Van Riel (2004) showed that animals with chronic hypercortisolism displayed an attenuation of 5HT1A-receptor mediated responses to serotonin and proposed that chronic hyperactivity of the HPA axis results in decreased serotonin responsiveness. This in turn could potentially lead to depressive symptoms, based on the monoamine hypothesis of depression (Hirschfeld, 2000).

Using a transgenic mouse line which overproduced corticotropin-releasing hormone (CRH), Groenink et al. (2002) found that long-term hypersecretion of CRH in the brain resulted in elevated basal plasma corticosterone concentrations, hypertrophy of the adrenal gland, and nonsuppression of dexamethasone, a state marker of depression. They concluded that these mice may model the dysregulation of the HPA axis observed in major depressive disorder (MDD).

Meditation, stress reduction, and self-management of depression

As such, it is hypothesized that the reduction of stress response could be a protective factor against the development and relapse of depression (Reno & Halaris, 1990; Hardy & Gorwood, 1993). Benson and colleagues characterized the widespread physiological changes brought on by meditation as the Relaxation Response (RR). They contend that by down-regulating the sympathetic nervous system, RR characterizes a hypo-metabolic state, which leads to a trophotropic or restorative response. The trophotropic response reverses the ergotropic response, also known as the fight or flight response, which stress produces. As we summarize below, this model has been supported in a wide body of literature on both novice and experienced mediators using a variety of meditation techniques.

Extensive studies have been conducted which show that Transcendental Meditation (TM) can bring about many physiological responses, including reduced respiratory rate, reduced skin conductance, and decreased total peripheral resistance, all changes which usually reflect diminished sympathetic tone (Barrows & Jacobs, 2002). There were also studies showing TM leads to alterations of stress-related hormones such as adrenocorticotropic hormone, cortisol, growth hormone, thyroid-stimulating hormone, dehydroepiandrosterone sulfate, prolactin, epinephrine, norepinephrine, and β-endorphins (Jevning et al., 1992). In a series of studies, Benson and his team demonstrated that the Relaxation Response (RR), a form of meditation that uses a set of simple instructions, results in measurable, predictable, and reproducible physiologic changes that include reductions in oxygen consumption, carbon dioxide production, respiratory rate, blood pressure, and arterial blood lactate (Benson et al., 1974; Wallace et al., 1971). Additional physiological characteristics include low-frequency heart rate oscillations (Peng et al., 2004) and reduced responsivity to plasma norepinephrine (Hoffman et al., 1982), both of which are compatible to a trophotropic or restorative response. Although the precise mechanisms by which the RR induces these physiological changes are not understood, it has been hypothesized that meditation stimulates production of nitric oxide, which plays a role in causing vascular dilatation and decreasing activation of the HPA axis (Benson et al., 1978; Stefano & Esch, 2005; Stefano et al., 2006).

In an example of studies that have demonstrated more specific responses to meditation, Benson's colleagues, Peng et al. (1999), showed that meditation techniques led to increased heart rate variability, a sign of adaptive response to stress, among the advanced practitioners of Kundalini Yoga. Kundalini Yoga is a form of yoga consisting of a number of bodily postures, expressive movements, and utterances. This type of yoga is practiced with the aim to cultivate character, practice breathing patterns, and promote concentration. Using functional brain mapping, Lazar et al. (2000) studied right-handed subjects who had practiced Kundalini meditation daily for at least 4 years and showed that the practice of meditation led to significant signal increases in multiple areas of the brain during meditation, including the dorsolateral prefrontal and parietal cortices, the hippocampus/parahippocampus, the temporal lobe, the pregenual anterior cingulated cortex striatum, and the pre- and post-central gyri. The researchers concluded that meditation activates neural structures involved in attention and control of the autonomic nervous system. Later, Lazar et al. (2005) studied 20 participants with extensive insight meditation experience, which involves focused attention to internal experiences. They found that, compared with their matched controls, the practitioners of meditation possessed thicker prefrontal cortices and right anterior insulae, areas of the brain that are associated with attention and interoceptive and sensory processing. From these results, Lazar and colleagues argued that the practice of meditation may increase cortical plasticity.

Davidson et al. (2003) compared meditators who participated in an 8-week program in mindfulness meditation to waitlisted controls in their brain electrical activity and immunological responses to influenza vaccine. They found that, compared with the controls, meditators had significant increases in antibody titers to influenza vaccine and significant increases in left-sided anterior activation in their brain electrical activity, a pattern previously associated with positive affect. In addition, the magnitude of increase in left-sided brain activation predicted the magnitude of antibody titer rise to the vaccine.

Although these studies did not target patients who suffer from depression, they have provided the evidence that the practice of meditation could have an overall protective effect on the practitioner, including the reduction of the biological effects from stress, a presumed precipitant of depression.

Possible psychological mechanisms

Contemporary interpretation of the effects of meditation emphasizes a variety of potential psychological benefits derived from its practice, including relaxation, exposure, desensitization, de-automatization, catharsis, and counter-conditioning (Murphy et al., 1997). Others have mentioned the gain of insight, self-monitoring, self-control, and self-understanding as outcomes (Baer, 2003). Two psychological mechanisms that have may be especially important in understanding how mediation may be helpful for depression are enhanced regulation of attention and de-identification with negative thoughts (Walsh & Shapiro, 2006).

The importance of negative thoughts on relapse of depression

The risk of relapse and recurrence in those who have had a past history of depression is very high, and those who treat depression are aware of the lower amount of triggering required for each subsequent depressive episode. For patients who have recovered from an episode of depression, a mood that is slightly more negative than usual can trigger a large amount of negative thoughts (e.g. "I am a failure," "I am weak," etc.), along with somatic symptoms of weakness, fatigue, or unexplained pain. Both the negative thoughts and concerns about the somatic sensations often seem out of proportion to the objective situation. Patients who believed they had successfully recovered may find themselves feeling back at square one and end up inside a destructive rumination loop that constantly asks: "What has gone wrong?," "Why is this happening to me?," and "Where will it all end?" Such ruminations frequently prolong and deepen the negative mood. This risk factor has been documented in a series of studies on cognitive reactivity conducted by Segal and colleagues (1999; 2006). In two studies, individuals successfully treated with either cognitive behavioral therapy (CBT) or pharmacotherapy were asked to complete a self-report measure of negative cognition before and after a negative mood induction to measure cognitive reactivity (Segal et al., 1999). The degree of cognitive reactivity predicted subsequent relapse.

The discovery that, even when people feel well, the link between negative moods and negative thoughts remains present and ready to be re-activated is of enormous importance. This means that in order to sustain one's recovery from depression, one has to learn how to keep mild states of depression from spiraling out of control. In order to effectively do this, those with depression have to learn how to respond differently to negative thoughts and sensations, which may be triggered by a negative mood state.

Decreasing negative thoughts by regulation of attention

In the context of depression, mindfulness meditation training has the goal of helping participants better regulate their attention to reduce ruminative preoccupation (Segal et al., 2002). This is consistent with the historical use of meditation for spiritual growth. For example, in several of the world's major religions, such as Christianity, Buddhism, and Taoism, people meditated in order to draw their attention away from the outside world (Arias et al., 2006). By not focusing their attention on the secular world, people who meditated facilitated bringing about personal change by suspending their habits of judging and interpreting, and by attending to the present moment without allowing oneself to be distracted by anxieties, fantasies, and memories. In this regard, meditation can be viewed as a systematic way of regulating one's attention. Recent studies have supported the notion that meditation training can help to enhance the regulation of attention (Jha et al., 2007; Tang et al., 2007).

Decreasing negative thoughts by disidentification

A second process is disidentification, the method whereby the mind only observes and ceases to identify with mental content such as thoughts, feelings, and images (Walsh & Shapiro, 2006). The heightened awareness brought about by meditation allows meditators to recognize and disidentify thoughts and emotions and to observe all experiences with calm and equanimity. Meditators can do this because they have developed a tranquil state of mind, which has variously been described as "transcendental consciousness," "Zen," and "divine apathy," among other terms (Feuerstein, 1996; Goleman, 1988; Schumacher & Woerner, 1989). This idea is also consistent with a proposed psychodynamic mechanism whereby the practice of paying attention to one's mind and body, such as in meditation, decreases the need for psychological defenses of repression and suppression, and increases the awareness of the subtle interplay of mind, body, and environment (Delmonte, 1989).

Similarities between meditation and CBT in distancing oneself from thoughts

In mindfulness meditation training for depression, patients are encouraged to take a "decentered" view of their depressogenic thoughts, seeing them as mental events rather than accurate reflections of reality or core aspects of their identity (Segal et al., 2002). There is significant similarity between the therapeutic elements of meditation and cognitive behavioral therapy (CBT), a psychotherapy technique proven to be effective for the treatment of depression. In both CBT and meditation, individuals are encouraged to distance themselves from their thoughts, a process referred to as "metacognitive awareness." In CBT, this is done in order to assess one's thoughts objectively and to test their validity. In contrast, in meditation, practitioners are encouraged to observe their thoughts and feelings with the goal of accepting them as they are without fighting them. Although the purpose of observing thoughts in CBT and meditation are quite different, there is evidence that patients with a history of depression develop metacognitive awareness both from CBT and training in mindfulness meditation (Teasdale et al., 2002).

Studies show meditation training reduces depression and other forms of psychological distress (e.g. anxiety) across populations

Research has provided evidence for the effectiveness of meditation practice in decreasing depression symptoms in both non-clinical populations and patients with medical conditions, leading to the facilitation of remission and prevention of relapse in patients with depressive disorders.

Effectiveness of meditation for non-clinical populations

In the West, meditation has been used more as a technique for stress management to achieve wellness than as a means of achieving spiritual goals. Two randomized controlled experimental studies are included here to provide the evidence on the effectiveness of meditation for non-clinical populations. Astin (1997) examined the effects of an 8-week stress reduction program, based on training in mindfulness meditation, on volunteers. He found that experimental subjects showed greater reductions in overall psychological symptomatology, greater increase in overall sense of control, and had higher scores on a measure of spiritual experiences. In a similar study, Shapiro et al. (1998) studied the short-term effects of an 8-week meditation-based stress reduction intervention on premedical and medical students. The participants who received the intervention, when compared with the waitlist controls, reported less state and trait anxiety, less overall psychological distress including depression, and increased spiritual experiences. These positive outcomes were replicated in the waitlisted control group when they received the intervention. However, the long-term effects of mindfulness training for this population remain unknown.

Effectiveness of meditation for medical patients

In a study to assess the effects of a mindfulness meditation-based stress reduction (MBSR) program on cancer outpatients, Speca et al. (2000) randomized ninety patients with different types and stages of cancer into an intervention group and a waitlisted control group. The intervention group met weekly for 1.5 hours for 7 weeks to meditate together and also individually practiced meditation at home. After the intervention, patients in the treatment group had significantly lower scores on their mood disturbance and on subscales of depression, anxiety, anger, and confusion and reported more vigor than control subjects. The treatment group also had fewer overall symptoms of stress and fewer cardiopulmonary and gastrointestinal symptoms. The researchers concluded that the meditation program was effective in decreasing mood disturbance and stress symptoms in patients with a wide variety of cancer diagnoses, stages of illness, and ages.

However, a systematic review of studies on the effectiveness of the MBSR program failed to support the findings of Speca et al. (2000). Toneatto and Nguyen (2007) reviewed 15 studies in which MBSR was administered to patients with mood disorders; patients with medical conditions such as pain, cancer, and heart disease; and non-clinical populations such as community samples and undergraduate students. They found that when active control groups were used, MBSR did not show an effect on depression or anxiety. In the same review, the authors also pointed out that adherence to the MBSR program was infrequently assessed, and where assessments did occur, the relation between practicing mindfulness and changes in depression and anxiety was equivocal.

In a recent self-controlled study, patients with chronic medical symptoms who went through a 12-week multimodal intervention group, which included Relaxation Response (RR) training, positive psychology, cognitive restructuring, and diet and exercise therapy, were shown to improve in depression, anxiety, somatization, stress management skills, spirituality, and a wide range of physical symptoms (Samuelson et al., in preparation). Although this was an observational study, it has provided support for the usefulness of the Relaxation Response (RR)–based multimodal intervention on patients with multiple somatic symptoms, a common and chronic condition in primary care clinics.

Effectiveness of meditation for reduction of depression symptoms in patients with anxiety disorders

Using an observational study design, Jon Kabat-Zinn and colleagues (1992) studied the effects of the Mindfulness-Based Stress Reduction and Relaxation Program (MBSR) on 22 patients with generalized anxiety disorder or panic disorder. They demonstrated that subjects had significant reductions in multiple measures of anxiety and depression during the program and 3 months after the program. Later, Miller et al. (1995) performed a 3-year follow-up of the 22 subjects and found the improvement in anxiety and depression, which resulted from the MBSR program, was maintained throughout and after a 3-year period.

Eppley et al. (1989) performed a meta-analysis to study the differential effects of different relaxation techniques on trait anxiety. They found that Transcendental Meditation (TM) had positive and moderate effect size (0.7) on trait anxiety, and progressive relaxation, biofeedback, and various other forms of meditation all had positive, but smaller effect sizes (0.28–0.4). However, meditation with a concentration focus did not have a positive effect size. Eppley et al. also reported that the population studied, the duration of study, the hours of instruction, and the attrition rate all influenced the effect size significantly.

Brooks and Scarano (1985) studied the effectiveness of TM in the treatment of Vietnam veterans who were having difficulty readjusting to civilian life as a result of having symptoms related to post-traumatic stress disorder (PTSD). They recruited 18 male Vietnam veterans who sought treatment at the Denver Veteran Center and randomized them to either TM program or a control group. The TM program group received an initial 4-day instruction period of 1.5 hours per day and weekly follow-up meetings over a 3-month period, and the control group received weekly psychotherapy sessions. They reported that the TM treatment group showed significant improvement in PTSD symptoms, anxiety, depression, alcohol consumption, insomnia, and family problems, while the control group showed no improvement in any of these measures. The researchers concluded that the TM program is a useful therapeutic modality for the treatment of PTSD, but acknowledged that the small sample size might limit generalizability of the study outcomes.

Studies applying meditation training as relapse prevention for people with a history of depression

Based on Jon Kabat-Zinn's Mindfulness-Based Stress Reduction Program, Zindel Segal, Mark Williams, and John Teasdale combined mindfulness and cognitive therapy to develop Mindfulness-Based Cognitive Therapy (MBCT). This form of cognitive therapy was developed with the aim of reducing relapse and recurrence of depression for people who are vulnerable to episodes of this disorder. Composed of meditation focused on simple breathing techniques and various yoga stretches, MBCT helps participants become more aware of the present moment with both their minds and bodies. Through a series of classes spanning 8 weeks and listening to tapes at home during this period, MBCT participants learn about and practice mindfulness meditation. The members of these classes are also educated about depression and learn several cognitive therapy exercises, which show how one's thoughts can affect one's feelings and highlight the best methods participants can use to help themselves when depression threatens to overwhelm them. The more structured exercises of MBCT make this form of therapy different from the mindfulness meditation that is normally taught at retreat centers. However, at the core of MBCT remains the tradition of mindfulness meditation, the meditative practice that has been taught for two and a half millennia.

MBCT helps its participants see the cognitive patterns of their minds more clearly and learn to recognize when their mood begins to turn negative. By doing so, this form of cognitive therapy helps stop the train of negative thoughts that may be triggered by a negative mood. Thus participants develop the ability to allow distressing mood, thoughts, and sensations to simply flow through their minds, without making themselves distraught. Having learned these skills, participants can then stay in touch with the present moment and not waste their time worrying uselessly about the past or the future.

In a study looking at the effectiveness of MBCT, Teasdale et al. (2000) reported a multicenter randomized clinical trial conducted in Toronto and at two sites in the United Kingdom (Cambridge and Bangor) where 145 participants were assigned to receive either treatment-as-usual (TAU), or, in addition to TAU, to receive eight classes of MBCT. All study participants had been free of symptoms of depression for at least 3 months and were not taking antidepressant medication when they started the study. However, these study subjects were known to be vulnerable to future episodes of depression because they had had at least two episodes in their past that met criteria for a major depressive episode, with the last episode having occurred within the past 2 years. Upon entering the study, all participants were categorized by their number of previous episodes of depression: two episodes only, or more than two episodes. After 8 weeks of MBCT, these subjects were followed-up for 12 months. The results showed that MBCT substantially reduced the risk of relapse in those who had three or more previous episodes of depression, specifically from 66% to 37%. For patients with only two previous episodes, MBCT did not reduce relapse/recurrence. These findings have been replicated by Ma and Teasdale (2004), who compared the outcomes of depressed patients treated with MBCT plus treatment as usual (TAU) to treatment with TAU only; they showed that MBCT is an effective and efficient way to prevent relapse/recurrence in recovered depressed patients with three or more previous episodes.

Essentially, these two studies (Ma & Teasdale, 2004; Teasdale et al., 2000) demonstrated that MBCT is a valuable enhancement to usual care in terms of relapse prevention among patients at high risk by virtue of their history of recurrent depression. To address the question of whether MBCT is equivalent to another active treatment, Kuyken and colleagues (2008) conducted a study comparing the efficacy of MBCT and maintenance antidepressant medication. Patients in this study were individuals with a history of three or more episodes of depression who were currently being treated with antidepressant medication and experiencing partial or full remission from the most recent episode of depression. Patients were randomly assigned to one of two conditions: (1) maintenance antidepressant medication, or (2) MBCT plus support to taper/discontinue antidepressants. Seventy-five percent of the participants in the MBCT group did discontinue medication within 6 months of finishing the 8-week MBCT program. At a 15-month follow-up assessment, relapse rates were comparable, with a trend towards lower rates of relapse in MBCT (47%) than in the maintenance antidepressant medication condition (60%). At the 15-month follow-up, compared with the medication group, the MCBT group had significantly lower rates of residual depression symptoms and psychiatric comorbidity, as well as higher levels of quality of life. These results suggest that at-risk patients may be able to effectively prevent depression relapse and enhance quality of life using mindfulness meditation as a self-management strategy even if they discontinue antidepressant medication.

Studies applying meditation as a treatment for current depression

Given the promising results of the MBCT in preventing future episodes of depression among recovered patients, researchers have been increasingly examining whether mindfulness training is effective as a treatment for individuals with current symptoms of depression. We discuss some of the initial promising findings. Later in this section, we review a separate body of literature examining yoga as a treatment for current depression.

Mindfulness training as an intervention for current depression

Building on the studies supporting the efficacy of applying MBCT when individuals have fully recovered, there is emerging evidence that mindfulness may hold promise for addressing residual symptoms of depression. A recent pilot study from our research group and our collaborators at the Massachusetts General Hospital speaks to the potential efficacy of mindfulness training for people with treatment-resistant depression (i.e. those who have residual symptoms despite an adequate course of antidepressant medication). The 8-week group intervention consisted of elements of MBCT and coping skills drawn from dialectical behavior therapy (Linehan, 1993), a treatment approach that heavily emphasizes mindfulness skills. Patients receiving the group intervention along with standard care showed greater symptom reduction than patients randomized to a standard care–only waitlist. In another study examining the effects of MBCT on residual symptoms of depression, Kingston and colleagues (2007) used a non-randomized design to compare symptom improvement in two groups of patients: those receiving usual care and those receiving MBCT plus usual care. The group receiving MBCT showed greater reduction in self-reported depression symptoms.

In addition, there are several papers published from open trials, which suggest that mindfulness treatment can be applied when individuals are symptomatic. Ramel and colleagues (2004) reported reduction in depression symptoms and depressive rumination among a mixed sample of psychiatric outpatients in a Veterans Affairs (VA) hospital system clinic, all of whom had a history of mood disorder. Mindfulness training was also included in an integrative treatment for depression called Exposure-Based Cognitive Therapy, which was developed by Adele Hayes and colleagues (2007). In this intervention, mindfulness is used to help individuals become more comfortable experiencing upsetting emotions, which is essential for the exposure portion of the intervention (Hayes & Feldman, 2004). Patients who completed this treatment have been found to show substantial decreases in depression (Hayes et al., 2007) and increases in self-reported mindfulness (Kumar et al., 2008).

Another recent pilot study examined the feasibility of introducing MBCT in primary care settings. Finucane and Mercer (2006) treated 13 primary care patients who had either active recurrent depression or recurrent anxiety and depression with the 8-week MBCT. They found that, after the intervention, the subjects' anxiety and depression symptoms improved, thus supporting the use of MBCT for the treatment of depression. However, due to the small sample size and the lack of a treatment control, these findings are considered preliminary at this stage.

Yoga meditation as an intervention for current depression

In addition to the aforementioned studies, there were several studies which focused specifically on the use of yoga for patients with current depression or history of depression. Khumar et al. (1993) treated a group of severely depressed female college students with Shavasana yoga, which is a series of postures intended to rejuvenate one's body, mind, and spirit by reducing stress and tension, and compared their outcomes to those of a no-treatment control group. They found that 64% of those who practiced Shavasana yoga improved in their depression symptoms, an outcome which was significantly better than that of the control group. Janakiramaiah et al. (2000) randomized 45 patients hospitalized for depression into three groups to receive electroconvulsive therapy (ECT), imipramine (150-mg daily oral dose), and daily, 45-minute sessions of Sudarshan Kriya Yoga (SKY), which involves rhythmic hyperventilation at different rates of breathing. They found that the ECT group had the best remission rate (93%), and the imipramine and SKY group had comparable (67% versus 73%) remission rates.

In reviewing the evidence on yoga intervention for treatment of depression, Pilkington et al. (2005) identified five randomized controlled trials, including the study by Janakiramaiah et al. (2000), and reported that all the five trials showed positive results. The researchers cautioned the interpretation of the study results because methodological details such as method of randomization, concealment of allocation, blinding of assessors, compliance, and attrition rates were missing in all the studies. In a more recent pilot study, Butler et al. (2008) randomized 46 individuals with long-term depressive disorders into three groups: yoga meditation and psychoeducation, hypnosis and psychoeducation, and psychoeducation alone as the control group. The study showed that significantly more yoga meditation participants experienced a remission than did controls at the 9-month follow-up, and that eight hypnosis group participants experienced a remission, although the difference from controls was not statistically significant. They concluded that both yoga meditation and hypnosis showed promise for treating low- to moderate-level depression.

Challenges and limitations for studies in meditation

In this chapter, while we have noted studies that support meditation as a means to reduce stress-related physiological changes, the exact mechanisms through which meditation influences the brain to alleviate depression remain unclear. The clinical studies on meditation face challenges similar to those faced by research in many mind/body therapies, the outcomes of which depend a lot on the individuals involved, how successful they are in mastering the self-regulatory techniques, and whether they are compliant with home practice assignments. Many of the earlier studies used small sample sizes and self-selected subjects, who could possess certain characteristics such as age, gender, health habits, and high expectancy for meditation effects, which might influence the outcomes of the studies. Furthermore, many studies followed an observational design and used subjects as their own controls. Thus the improvements that were seen at the end simply could have resulted due to the lapse of time. As reported by Toneatto and Nguyen (2007), many studies, which applied more stringent research designs such as including use of active control groups, failed to show positive effects of meditation.

In addition, there have been relatively few randomized controlled trials on a well-defined population of subjects with depression. Although the two MBCT relapse prevention studies (Teasdale et al., 2000; Ma & Teasdale, 2004) are quite positive, there are several limitations worth noting (Coelho et al., 2007). First, MBCT seems to only prevent relapses in individuals with three or more previous episodes of depression. Thus this leaves open the question of whether MBCT would be useful for individuals with two or less episodes. Second, the relapse prevention studies of MBCT did not employ an active comparison treatment in addition to usual care, making it difficult to attribute treatment effects specifically to MBCT, rather than simply benefits of receiving any intervention in addition to usual care. The more recent study by Kuyken and colleagues (2008) reviewed above begins to address this question by demonstrating that MBCT may be equivalent – and in some cases superior – to maintenance antidepressant medication as a relapse prevention strategy.

Thus far, neither MBCT nor any other form of meditation has been proven as an effective stand-alone treatment for current depression. The studies on yoga meditation indicated that yoga could be a promising treatment for current depression. However, these studies did not report adequately on concealment of allocation, blinding of assessors, and compliance and attrition of the participants. Despite the significant limitations that exist in the available evidence, the use of meditation continues to have its appeals for calming and regulating the moods of people with depression. Rather than using meditation as the sole treatment for depression, current evidence supports its use as an adjunct therapy in the treatment of depression and for prevention of relapse among those who have had multiple episodes of depression in the past. However, there is evidence that recovered patients may be able to safely discontinue antidepressant medication following participation in an MBCT program (Kuyken et al., 2008).

Practical considerations: how to refer patients to meditation training?

As we discussed earlier in this chapter, meditation may reduce stress, anxiety, and depression, and at the same time, may enhance empathy, life satisfaction, and self-compassion (Shapiro et al., 1998). Due to all of these positive effects, meditation is gaining popularity and acceptance as a health practice to manage one's mood so one can enjoy tranquillity, self-acceptance, and self-actualization.

Clinicians may encourage interested patients to explore meditation as a method for stress reduction and self-regulation of mood symptoms and to augment conventional psychopharmacological and psychotherapeutic treatments of depression. In the following sections, we present some practical recommendations for integrating meditation into a treatment plan for patients with depression.

To whom should you recommend meditation?

There is limited research to date in terms of which patients with depression would benefit from meditation. The most conservative recommendation informed by published literature (Kuyken et al., 2008; Teasdale et al., 2000; Ma & Teasdale, 2004) would be to introduce meditation training as a relapse prevention strategy for individuals who have recovered from depression. Again, based on the literature, this approach would be expected to be most effective for individuals with highly recurrent depression (three or more previous episodes). However, the clinical reality is that many clinicians will have contact with individuals who are currently experiencing depression. Is there any harm in introducing meditation training when individuals are currently depressed?

As described in our literature review, there is growing evidence that meditation may be successfully introduced to individuals who are currently depressed as a component of psychotherapy. However, although meditation can have a stabilizing effect for individuals with current depression, it may also have a destabilizing effect as individuals come into contact with upsetting thoughts and memories (Hayes & Feldman, 2004). As with most treatment methods, meditation may produce side effects or complications for some of its practitioners. For beginners, meditation may evoke traumatic memories or existential anxieties, which, though distressing, are usually mild and transient (Germer et al., 2005). Occasionally, severe anxiety and hallucinatory experiences may arise. However, this occurs more frequently in practitioners with prior severe pathology who are involved in intensive meditative retreats (Walsh & Vaughan, 1993). If approached skillfully, many of these complications can be used as opportunities for learning or healing, particularly if meditation teachers or psychotherapists with meditation experience are available to provide proper guidance to these beginners. Indeed, this contact with upsetting material during meditation is consistent with the goals of exposure-based psychotherapies that have been shown to be highly effective for anxiety disorders (Baer, 2003; Hayes & Feldman, 2004; Roemer & Orsillo, 2007).

Naturally, caution is appropriate in referring meditation to patients with a history of psychotic symptoms, current suicidal ideation, and severe unresolved trauma. However, brief meditation exercises are included as a component of treatment for individuals with severe psychopathology such as dialectical behavior therapy, a treatment for patients with borderline personality disorder who often present with one or more of these symptoms (Linehan, 1993). Nonetheless, if a clinician is concerned about potential adverse reactions to meditation, several steps may be taken to help increase the likelihood of success. First, it may be useful to recommend that meditation training be undertaken in a structured manner from either a meditation teacher or psychotherapist who has experience integrating meditation into treatment. Such a professional could help to customize training to address any challenges the patient presents in terms of motivational deficits and would be able to respond appropriately to any adverse reactions. Second, for patients with difficulties with concentration, it may also be useful to recommend home practice materials that include guided audio recordings. Third, it may be helpful to recommend gradually increasing the length of meditation practice from a few minutes a day before building to the 20- to 45-minute sessions recommended in some programs. Fourth, it may also be helpful to consider more active forms of meditation as an alternative to sitting forms of meditation. As we reported earlier in this chapter, there is considerable evidence that yoga can be effective in reducing symptoms of depression. Such an approach may help to increase awareness of somatic experience, which may be a useful precursor to the potentially more challenging task of observing thoughts involved in sitting meditation. In addition, yoga may also offer many of the same benefits described in the chapter on physical exercise.

A final consideration is the degree of cost associated with meditation training. Some training programs may represent a significant investment for some patients. For patients of limited economic means, there are a few options. The self-help resources recommended in Appendix A are one cost-effective alternative for gaining an introduction to meditation techniques. Another option to explore with patients would be learning meditation through stress-management programs offered in workplaces or at various places in their communities, such as hospitals or other health care facilities, which may be covered by the patient's insurance plan.

Role of the clinician

The role of the clinician will vary considerably. At a minimum, the clinician may be the individual who recommends that the patient pursue meditation and provide concrete suggestions on how to learn more about it. Appendix A provides a list of self-instructional resources (books and audio-recordings) as well as links to websites where patients can locate a meditation teacher. At the other end of the continuum, depending on their level of training and experience, the clinician may provide instruction in meditation themselves. How much training and experience a clinician needs likely varies. At one extreme, advocates of Transcendental Meditation (TM) purport that it can only be taught effectively by a certified trainer (Roth, 1994). The developers of MBCT recommend that anyone providing mindfulness training for depression should currently be practicing meditation (Segal et al., 2002). On the one hand, such personal experience as a teacher enhances creditability and competence, allows for modeling of the attitudes and behaviors associated with meditation practice, and provides insights that may be useful to effectively troubleshoot challenges that arise for patients as they are learning to meditate. On the other hand, overly rigid practice and training requirements may limit the degree to which basic meditation techniques can be disseminated. For this reason, as noted earlier, the techniques in Benson's *Relaxation Response* (1975) are relatively easy to learn, and most clinicians with experience in teaching stress management will likely feel comfortable teaching these techniques to patients.

In summary, the degree of training a clinician requires in order to teach meditation likely depends on the complexity of the techniques being taught. As a final thought, it is worth noting that acquiring qualifications and expertise are not the only reasons a clinician should consider learning to meditate. Meditation may also be an approach that health professionals can use to take better care of themselves, perhaps leading them to provide care with more empathy and compassion.

How to introduce meditation

Some patients may be more open to trying mediation than others. Given increased coverage of meditation in the popular media, the number of people willing to try it is likely increasing. However, some patients may carry perceptions that meditation is too exotic or foreign for their comfort. As such, it may be more helpful to focus on phrases that may be less loaded for some than "meditation," such as "relaxation," "stress management," or "coping skills." Others may worry that practicing these techniques, which have their roots in Eastern spiritual practice, will contradict their religious beliefs. As such, it may be helpful to explain that meditation can be practiced in a manner that does not contradict other religious practices. Indeed, the approaches recommended in Appendix A are all presented from a secular perspective. As a different approach, patients with strong religious orientation may be encouraged to discuss meditation with their clergy to learn about meditation traditions within their particular faith.

Enhancing motivation

Meditation, like any lifestyle modification, can be hard to integrate into a person's day-to-day routine for regular practice. As such, many of the techniques described in the chapter on exercise will apply here. It may be useful to create a list of pros and cons for both meditation and continuing not to meditate. Helping the patient find his or her own motivation will ultimately be the most important step. Time management can also be a barrier to regular meditation practice. For patients who report having no time to meditate, it may be useful to begin with brief meditation exercises or encourage the patient to try exchanging meditation for some other regular activity used for relaxation, such as watching television. Patients with little structure to their daily routine can be encouraged to schedule meditation at a time of day when they will be sufficiently alert.

Summary and conclusion

Meditation has been used for several millennia to cultivate calmness, concentration, and positive emotions in many cultures. It has the promise to be even more fully integrated into conventional medicine to serve as an important self-management skill for the management of depression and for preventing relapse of depression. There is evidence to show that meditation brings about a hypometabolic state which counteracts the physiological changes triggered by stress. Meditation may alleviate depression through reduction of stress responses, enhanced regulation of attention, and de-identification with negative thoughts. Meditation has been shown to be effective for reducing the risk of relapse among those who had three or more previous episodes of depression. Preliminary data suggest that meditation, including yoga, may also be potentially useful for treating patients with current depression. Clinicians may play an important role by understanding and even advocating the use of meditation as a skill for self-management to augment conventional psychopharmacological and psychotherapeutic treatments of depression. Interested readers are encouraged to use the information listed in Appendix A to find the resources to learn more about meditation.

REFERENCES

Abelson JL, Khan S, Liberzon I, Young EA. HPA axis activity in patients with panic disorder: review and synthesis of four studies. *Depress Anxiety.* 2007; 24(1):66–76.

Arias AJ, Steinberg K, Banga A, Trestman RL. Systematic review of the efficacy of meditation techniques as treatment for medical illness. *J Altern Complement Med.* 2006; 12(8):817–832.

Astin J. Stress reduction through mindfulness meditation. *Psychother Psychosom.* 1997; 66:97–106.

Astin JA, Shapiro SL, Eisenberg DM, Forys KL. Mind-body medicine: state of the science, implications for practice. *J Am Board Fam Pract.* 2003; 16:131–147.

Baer R. Mindfulness training as a clinical intervention: a conceptual and empirical review. *Clin Psychol Sci Pract.* 2003; 10:125–143.

Barrows KA, Jacobs BP. Mind-body medicine. An introduction and review of the literature. *Med Clin North Am.* 2002; 86(1):11–31.

Benson, H. *The Relaxation Response.* New York, NY: HarperCollins Publishers; 1975.

Benson H, Beary JF, Carol MP. The relaxation response. *Psychiatry.* 1974; 37:37–46.

Benson H, Dryer T, Hartley LH. Decreased VO2 consumption during exercise with elicitation of the relaxation response. *J Hum Stress.* 1978; 4(2):38–42.

Brooks JS, Scarano T. Transcendental Meditation in the treatment of post-Vietnam adjustment. *J Couns Dev.* 1985; 64:212–215.

Butler LD, Waelde LC, Hastings TA, Chen XH, Symons B, Marshall J, Kaufman A, Nagy TF, Blasey CM, Seibert EO, Spiegel D. Meditation with yoga, group therapy with hypnosis, and psychoeducation for long-term depressed mood: a randomized pilot trial. *J Clin Psychol.* 2008; 64(7):806–820.

Coelho HF, Canter PH, Ernst E. Mindfulness-based cognitive therapy: evaluating current evidence and informing future research. *J Consult Clin Psychol.* 2007; 75(6):1000–1005.

Collins C. Yoga: intuition, preventive medicine, and treatment. *J Obstet Gynecol Neonatal Nurs.* 1998; 27(5):563–568.

Davidson RJ, Kabat-Zinn J, Schumacher J, Rosenkranz M, Muller D, Santorelli SF, Urbanowski F, Harrington A, Bonus K, Sheridan JF. Alternations in brain and immune function produced by mindfulness meditation. *Psychosom Med.* 2003; 65(4): 564–570.

Delmonte MM. Meditation, the unconscious, and psychosomatic disorders. *Int J Psychosom.* 1989; 36(1–4):45–52.

Eppley KR, Abrams AI, Shear J. Differential effects of relaxation techniques on trait anxiety: a meta-analysis. *J Clin Psychol.* 1989; 45(6):957–974.

Feuerstein G. *The Shambhala Guide to Yoga.* Boston, MA: Shambhala; 1996.

Finucane A, Mercer SW. An exploratory mixed methods study of the acceptability and effectiveness of Mindfulness-Based Cognitive Therapy for patients with active depression and anxiety in primary care. *BMC Psychiatry.* 2006; 7:6–14.

Germer CK, Siegel RD, Fulton PR. *Mindfulness and Psychotherapy.* New York, NY: Guilford Press; 2005.

Goleman D. *The Meditative Mind.* New York, NY: J.P. Tarcher; 1988.

Groenink L, Dirks A, Verdouw PM, Schipholt M, Veening JG, van Der Gugten J, Olivier B. HPA axis dysregulation in mice overexpressing corticotropin releasing hormone. *Biol Psychiatry.* 2002; 51(11):875–881.

Hardy P, Gorwood P. Impact of life events in the course of depression. *Encephale.* 1993; 19(3):481–489.

Hayes AM, Feldman G. Clarifying the construct of mindfulness in the context of emotion regulation and the process of change in therapy. *Clin Psychol Sci Pract.* 2004; 11(3):255–262.

Hayes AM, Feldman GC, Beevers CG, Laurenceau JP, Cardaciotto L, Lewis-Smith J. Discontinuities and cognitive changes in an exposure-based cognitive therapy for depression. *J Consult Clin Psychol.* 2007; 75(3):409–421.

Hirschfeld RM. History and evolution of the monoamine hypothesis of depression. *J Clin Psychiatry.* 2000; 61(Suppl 6):4–6.

Hoffman JW, Benson H, Arns PA, Stainbrook GL, Landsberg GL, Young JB, Gill A. Reduced sympathetic nervous system responsivity associated with the relaxation response. *Science.* 1982; 215(4529):190–192.

Janakiramaiah N, Gangadhar BN, Naga Venkatesha Murthy PJ, Harish MG, Subbakrishna DK, Vedamurthachar A. Antidepressant efficacy of Sudarshan Kriya Yoga (SKY) in melancholia: a randomized comparison with electroconvulsive therapy (ECT) and imipramine. *J Affect Disord.* 2000; 57(1–3):255–259.

Jevning R, Wallace RK, Beidebach M. The physiology of meditation: a review. A wakeful hypometabolic integrated response. *Neurosci Biobehav Rev.* 1992; 16(3):415–424.

Jha AP, Krompinger J, Baime MJ. Mindfulness training modifies subsystems of attention. *Cogn Affect Behav Neurosci.* 2007; 7(2):109–119.

Kabat-Zinn, J. *Full Catastrophe Living: Using the Wisdom of Your Body and Mind to Face Stress, Pain, and Illness.* New York, NY: Delacorte Press; 1990.

Kabat-Zinn J, Massion AO, Kristeller J, Peterson LG, Fletcher KE, Pbert L, Lenderking WR, Santorelli SF. Effectiveness of a meditation-based stress reduction program in the treatment of anxiety disorders. *Am J Psychiatry.* 1992; 149(7):936–943.

Kingston T, Dooley B, Bates A, Lawlor E, Malone K. Mindfulness-based cognitive therapy for residual depressive symptoms. *Psychol Psychother.* 2007; 80(Pt 2):193–203.

Khumar SS, Kaur P, Kaur S. Effectiveness of Shavasana on depression among university students. *Indian J Clin Psychol.* 1993; 20:82–87.

Kumar SM, Feldman GC, Hayes AM. Change in mindfulness and emotion regulation in an exposure-based cognitive therapy for depression. *Cognit Ther Res.* 2008; 32:734–744.

Kuyken W, Byford S, Taylor RS, Watkins E, Holen E, White K, et al. Mindfulness-based cognitive therapy to prevent relapse in recurrent depression. *J Consult Clin Psychol.* 2008; 76:966–978.

Lazar SW, Bush G, Gollub RL, Fricchione GL, Khalsa G, Benson H. Functional brain mapping of the relaxation response and meditation. *Neuroreport.* 2000; 11(7):1581–1585.

Lazar SW, Kerr CE, Wasserman RH, Gray JR, Greve DN, Treadway MT, McGarvey M, Quinn BT, Dusek JA, Benson H, Rauch SL, Moore CI, Fischl B. Meditation experience is associated with increased cortical thickness. *Neuroreport.* 2005; 16(17):1893–1897.

Linehan MM. Dialectical behavior therapy for treatment of borderline personality disorder: implications for the treatment of substance abuse. *NIDA Res Monogr.* 1993; 137:201–216.

Ma SH, Teasdale JD. Mindfulness-based cognitive therapy for depression: replication and exploration of differential relapse prevention effects. *J Consult Clin Psychol.* 2004; 72(1):31–40.

Mahesh, MY. *The Science of Being and Art of Living: Transcendental Meditation.* Delhi, India: Maharishi's Publication; 1963 (first publication); Plume; 2001 (reprint).

Miller J, Fletcher K, Kabat-Zinn J. Three-year follow-up and clinical implications of a mindfulness meditation-based stress reduction intervention in the treatment of anxiety disorders. *Gen Hosp Psychiatry.* 1995; 17(3):192–200.

Murphy, Michael, Donovan, Steven and Eugene Taylor. *The Physical and Psychological Effects of Meditation: A Review of Contemporary Research with a Comprehensive Bibliography.* 2nd edn. Petaluma, CA: Institute of Noetic Sciences; 1997.

Pariante CM. Depression, stress and the adrenal axis. *J Neuroendocrinol.* 2003; 15(8):811–812.

Peng CK, Mietus JE, Liu Y, Khalsa G, Douglas PS, Benson H, Goldberger AL. Exaggerated heart rate oscillations during two meditation techniques. *Int J Cardiol.* 1999; 70(2):101–107.

Peng CK, Henry IC, Mietus JE, Hausdorff JM, Khalsa G, Benson H, Goldberger AL. Heart rate dynamics during three forms of meditation. *Int J Cardiol.* 2004; 95(1):19–27.

Pilkington K, Kirkwood G, Rampes H. Yoga for depression: the research evidence. *J Affect Disord.* 2005; 89(1–3):13–24.

Ramel W, Goldin PR, Carmona PE, McQuaid JR. The effects of mindfulness meditation on cognitive processes and affect in patients with past depression. *Cognit Ther Res.* 2004; 28(4):433–455.

Reno RM, Halaris AE. The relationship between life stress and depression in an endogenous sample. *Compr Psychiatry.* 1990; 31(1):25–33.

Roemer L, Orsillo SM. An open trial of an acceptance-based behavior therapy for generalized anxiety disorder. *Behav Ther.* 2007; 38(1):78–85.

Roth R. *Maharishi Mahesh Yogi's Transcendental Meditation.* Washington, DC: Primus; 1994.

Schumacher S, Woerner G (eds). *The Encyclopedia of Eastern Philosophy and Religion*. Boston, MA: Shambhala; 1989.

Segal ZV, Gemar M, Williams S. Differential cognitive response to a mood challenge following successful cognitive therapy or pharmacotherapy for unipolar depression. *J Abnorm Psychol*. 1999; 108(1):3–10.

Segal ZV, Teasdale JD, Williams JM. *Mindfulness-Based Cognitive Therapy for Depression*. New York, NY: Guilford Press; 2002.

Segal ZV, Kennedy S, Gemar M, Hood K, Pedersen R, Buis T. Cognitive reactivity to sad mood provocation and the prediction of depressive relapse. *Arch Gen Psychiatry*. 2006; 63(7):749–755.

Shapiro S, Schwarz G, Bonner G. Effects of mindfulness-based stress reduction on medical and premedical students. *J Behav Med*. 1998; 21:581–599.

Speca M, Carlson L, Goodney E, Angen M. A randomized, wait-list controlled clinical trial: the effect of a mindfulness meditation-based stress reduction program on mood and symptoms of stress in cancer outpatients. *Psychsom Med*. 2000; 62(5):613–622.

Stefano GB, Esch T. Integrative medical therapy: examination of meditation's therapeutic and global medicinal outcomes via nitric oxide. *Int J Mol Med*. 2005; 16(4):621–630.

Stefano GB, Fricchione GL, Esch T. Relaxation: molecular and physiological significance. *Med Sci Monit*. 2006; 12(9):HY21–31.

Swaab DF, Bao AM, Lucassen PJ. The stress system in the human brain in depression and neurodegeneration. *Ageing Res Rev*. 2005; 4(2):141–194.

Tang YY, Ma Y, Wang J, Fan Y, Feng S, Lu Q, Yu Q, Sui D, Rothbart MK, Fan M, Posner MI. Short-term meditation training improves attention and self-regulation. *Proc Natl Acad Sci USA*. 2007; 104(43):17152–17156.

Teasdale JD, Segal ZV, Williams JMG, Ridgeway V, Lau M, Soulsby J. Reducing risk of recurrence of major depression using Mindfulness-based Cognitive Therapy. *J Consult Clin Psychol*. 2000; 68:615–623.

Teasdale JD, Moore RG, Hayhurst H, Pope M, Williams S, Segal ZV. Metacognitive awareness and prevention of relapse in depression: empirical evidence. *J Consult Clin Psychol*. 2002; 70(2):275–287.

Toneatto T, Nguyen L. Does mindfulness meditation improve anxiety and mood symptoms? A review of the controlled research. *Can J Psychiatry*. 2007; 52(4):260–266.

Van Riel, E. Dysregulation of the HPA-axis: implications for serotonin responses in the hippocampus. Doctoral dissertation, Universiteit van Amsterdam, 2004. Available at http://dare.uva.nl/record/161039

Wallace KR, Benson H, Wilson AF. A wakeful hypometabolic physiologic state. *Am J Physiol*. 1971; 221:795–799.

Walsh R, Shapiro SL. The meeting of meditative disciplines and Western Psychology: a mutually enriching dialogue. *Am Psychol*. 2006; 61(3):227–239.

Walsh R, Vaughan F. *Paths Beyond Ego: The Transpersonal Vision*. Los Angeles, CA: Tarcher; 1993.

Yehuda R, Giller EL, Southwick SM, Lowy MT, Mason JW. Hypothalamic-pituitary-adrenal dysfunction in posttraumatic stress disorder. *Biol Psychiatry*. 1991; 30(10):1031–1048.

Appendix A   Resources for learning about meditation

Meditation can be an effective way for managing stress, reducing anxiety and depression symptoms, and developing greater personal awareness. There is also evidence that meditation training may help you manage depression by helping to prevent relapse. The purpose of this hand-out is to provide an introductory list of resources to help you learn meditation techniques. We should note that there are many different types of meditation and methods for learning how to meditate. Indeed, various forms of meditation have been practiced across cultures for centuries. In the list below, we have focused on approaches that have been widely researched and have been demonstrated to promote various aspects of mental and physical health. However, we also acknowledge that no one approach is appropriate for all. As such, we also encourage you to explore other approaches to meditation that may be more consistent with your culture, lifestyle, values, or beliefs.

Mindfulness-based stress reduction (MBSR)

Jon Kabat-Zinn's *Full Catastrophe Living* (1990; New York: Delacorte) describes the Mindfulness-Based Stress Reduction (MBSR) program in a very engaging manner. Audio recordings of guided meditation lead by Kabat-Zinn are available at www.stressreductiontapes.com. For more information about learning MBSR from a teacher, visit www.umassmed.edu/cfm.

Mindfulness-based cognitive therapy for depression (MBCT)

This approach is specifically designed to help manage depression. It combines techniques from mindfulness-based stress reduction (MBCT) and cognitive behavioral psychotherapy. In research studies, it is typically taught in an 8-week class. A recent book by the creators of this program is available to introduce the basic concepts and techniques: *The Mindful Way Through Depression: Freeing Yourself From Chronic Unhappiness* (2007; New York: Guildford Press). This book also comes with a CD of several guided meditation exercises. For more information on learning MBCT, visit www.mbct.com.

The Relaxation Response (RR)

Herbert Benson's *The Relaxation Response* (1975; William Morrow and Company, Inc.), introduces simple and easy-to-learn techniques on relaxation and meditation. For more information on learning these techniques, visit www.mbmi.org.

Transcendental Meditation (TM)

Transcendental Meditation (TM) was introduced by Maharishi Mahesh Yogi in the late 1950s. TM is a technique practiced twice daily for 15 to 20 minutes. Robert Roth's *Maharishi Mahesh Yogi's Transcendental Meditation* (1994; Washington, DC: Primus) provides an enthusiastic introduction to this approach. For more information about learning TM, visit www.tm.org.

Cultivating social support

The role of peer support in self-management

Social isolation and lack of social support increases the risk of developing depression and may prolong episodes of depression (Brown & Harris, 1978; Joiner, 1997; Kendler et al., 2005; Sherbourne et al., 1995). As such, peer support interventions are a logical component of self-management for depression. Peer support interventions for medical and psychiatric disorders exist to provide members with the opportunity to give and receive emotional support, information about disorders and their treatment, and encouragement in coping with the disorder itself and adhering to treatment. The peer who provides the support is typically an individual who has previously had first-hand experience with the condition. The format for the support can include group or individual interventions. Peer support groups have traditionally involved face-to-face meetings but are increasingly available via telephone- or Internet-based communications.

In this chapter, we discuss how peer support interventions are relevant to the goals of self-management, review the growing body of research examining the utility and efficacy of peer-led support interventions, and discuss practical considerations for integrating peer support interventions into a treatment plan. As part of the section on practical considerations, we will also address resources for family and friends of individuals with depression, as well as resources to help individuals with depression enhance their social skills as a means of protecting and strengthening existing relationships.

The role of peer support in self-management

Peer support interventions are a key component of the Chronic Care Model (Wagner et al., 1998), a self-management model of chronic disease discussed in Chapter 1. Peer support interventions are consistent with several goals of self-management. By definition, these interventions are delivered by peers or other non-professionals (also referred to as paraprofessionals), which is in keeping with the goal of reducing reliance on contact with a clinician for treatment. Indeed, various forms of peer support interventions are sometimes referred to as "self-help" interventions, although "mutual help" may be a more accurate description. Discussions with peers can reinforce psychoeducational information about depression introduced elsewhere in the self-management treatment plan and can underscore the importance of adherence to treatment goals. Through peer-to-peer feedback and coaching on effective communication with clinicians, peer support interventions can also enhance the collaborative relationship between patients and clinicians that is central to self-management. Given that many patients with depression may be socially isolated, attending a peer support intervention may even be conceptualized as a lifestyle modification. Also, the regularity and relatively high frequency of contact with peers may facilitate self-monitoring, which may lead to earlier professional interventions as symptoms begin to worsen, thereby reducing the risk of relapse or need for hospitalization.

Peer support may also uniquely contribute to the development of patient self-efficacy (Bandura, 1997), a key component of self-management. Peers who are successfully coping with depression may serve as role models of disease management and increase other patients' confidence that their own behavior changes will result in wellness. Stated differently, interactions with higher-functioning peers who acknowledge past struggles may provide hope for lower-functioning individuals that progress and stabilization are possible (Sheffield, 2003).

Research on peer support for depression and other disorders

Across disorders, peer support is widely used and acceptable to patients. Nearly one fifth of US adults report attending at least one self-help group meeting at some point in their lifetime, and 3% to 4% participate in a given year (Kessler et al., 1997). Participants frequently evaluate self-help groups as being as effective as psychotherapy (Seligman, 1995). Individuals with more stigmatizing conditions are more likely to seek out support groups than those with less "embarrassing" conditions (Davison et al., 2000), making them especially relevant for depression.

Peer support has been studied in a variety of formats to address a variety of conditions using a range of research designs. As such, systematic reviews reveal that peer support interventions for various medical and psychiatric disorders presented in both face-to-face (Hogan et al., 2002) and Internet-based (Eysenbach et al., 2004) formats may be helpful in decreasing symptoms of depression and increasing social support, but acknowledge that limitations in study designs preclude more definitive conclusions. A frequent limitation is that peer support is rarely evaluated in isolation (Eysenbach et al., 2004), but instead it is typically studied as part of a comprehensive intervention involving professionally delivered interventions. Similarly, a recent review of randomized controlled studies of paraprofessional-delivered interventions for depression and anxiety concluded that these interventions are superior to no treatment, but it was not possible to determine whether these interventions were comparable to professionally delivered interventions (den Boer et al., 2005). This issue is of somewhat less concern within the self-management approach, where peer support is used to augment professionally delivered interventions. Nonetheless, it does present challenges in determining their effectiveness.

Given that it is difficult to make generalized statements about peer support interventions, our literature review will focus on high-quality studies of both face-to-face and telephone- and Internet-based interventions where depression is the primary treatment target. Given that the involvement of non-professionals in delivering these interventions may lessen the confidence of some clinicians (Powell et al, 2000b; Salzer et al., 1999) as well as patients, we will give particular attention in this review to the types of training given to paraprofessionals and evidence of their effectiveness. After discussing the promise and potential limitations of peer-led support groups, we conclude the review with a discussion of factors that emerged across studies that may help lead to optimal performance of peer-led interventions. We will review three types of studies: peer-led support groups, individual peer support, and Internet-based peer support interventions.

Studies of peer-led support groups

One of the most rigorous studies of examining the efficacy of group interventions led by paraprofessionals was conducted by Bright et al., (1999). Briefly, this study compared two 10-week interventions which met for 90-minute sessions: (1) cognitive behavioral therapy (CBT; a structured group intervention focused on teaching participants to identify, dispute, and correct distorted thinking and dysfunctional beliefs through group exercises and supplemental reading of *Feeling Good* as a form of bibliotherapy) and (2) mutual support group (a less structured group in which group leaders facilitate the development of interpersonal insight, the acquisition of disclosure skills, and the sharing of feedback and advice among members). Each intervention was delivered by either a professional (Master's level psychologist) or paraprofessional (individuals recruited from community-based self-help groups with no post-baccalaureate mental health–related degree or experience administering individual psychotherapy). Both professionals and paraprofessionals received 3 days of training in both CBT and mutual support and led each type of group at least once in the study. Participants in the study were randomly assigned to one of four groups: CBT led by two professionals, CBT led by two paraprofessionals, mutual support led by two professionals, or mutual support led by two paraprofessionals. In general, participants in all four conditions demonstrated comparable rates of clinical significant improvement (defined as a large reduction in depression symptoms). The professional therapists achieved slightly better results than the paraprofessionals in terms of producing remission of symptoms, but this was only true in the CBT condition. In other words, both professionals and paraprofessionals achieved similar levels of achieving remission when leading mutual support groups. These results suggest that although CBT may be optimally delivered by trained professional therapists, paraprofessionals leading mutual support interventions can help to achieve clinically meaningful improvements in depression symptoms and are equally as effective as professional therapists.

A second recent study tested a cognitive self-therapy (CST; den Boer et al., 2006) which involved a blend of professional- and peer-delivered interventions. In this program, patients are given a manual to learn techniques for restructuring cognitive schema by focusing on problems in interpersonal functioning and initially attend group sessions led by a nurse, social worker, or psychologist to learn and practice cognitive restructuring skills. Once patients have learned these skills, they have the option of receiving further training to be able to lead CST self-therapy meetings with other patients. In other words, the patients evolve into peer counselors. In a recent randomized controlled trial of patients with chronic anxiety and depressive disorders (den Boer et al., 2006), participants in the CST condition were found to have less medical treatment utilization (therapist contact and hospitalizations) than a treatment-as-usual group receiving professionally delivered individual psychotherapy. Consistent with the goals of self-management, a skills-based peer-led intervention may help reduce utilization of professional services. Interestingly, the CST group showed similar degrees of improvement in depression symptoms as the comparison group. This equivalence in outcomes between professionally delivered individual psychotherapy and group-based, self-administered treatment with minimal clinician involvement has considerable implications, given the latter holds promise as being a less costly treatment option. As we will discuss in a later section, the authors caution that a program like CST would tend to be most appropriate for highly motivated patients, as reflected by relatively low rates of treatment adherence.

A third study showing promise for peer-led interventions is a recently published pilot study testing a peer-led chronic disease self-management group combined with telephone-based care management (see description of this approach in Chapter 2) in a sample of individuals with chronic depression (Ludman et al., 2007). In this study, group leaders were non-professionals who completed a 4-day training period and used a highly structured manual to lead the groups. The manual is not specific to depression but rather addresses several skill areas relevant to coping with any chronic disease, including disease-related problem solving, symptom management (e.g. relaxation), and communication with clinicians. The program consisted of a structured 6-week program supplemented with bi-monthly meetings using a structured method for group problem solving and action planning. Group leaders received occasional supervision by a study psychologist. The study compared four conditions: (1) the combination of care-management and peer-led groups as described above, (2) care-management plus professionally led CBT group (10 weeks plus twice-monthly booster sessions), (3) a care-management-only group, and (4) a treatment-as-usual control group. In this study, patients were recruited from a behavioral health clinic that is part of a large health maintenance organization (HMO) and were free to use any other forms of non-study treatment normally available. Although patients in all four study conditions showed improvement in depression symptoms, the peer-led group was not superior to any of the other three treatment approaches; however, the authors caution that the study's sample size may have been too small to detect small effects. Far fewer of the peer-led group members attended follow-up sessions than did members of the professionally led CBT group. This result suggests that peer-led interventions may be as effective in terms of reducing symptoms as professionally led groups; however, this particular peer-led intervention may need to be refined to enhance retention and patient satisfaction.

Two interesting observations by the researchers may help inform more effective future interventions. First, patients expressed some dissatisfaction with the "generic" self-management intervention used in the peer-led groups. Use of such generic protocols may hold promise for treating mixed groups with a variety of chronic diseases (thus increasing the availability of such interventions and potentially decreasing stigma by treating depression as comparable to other chronic medical conditions). However, patients expressed interest in more depression-specific content in the group. A second qualitative finding was that many of the members of the professionally led CBT group continued to meet for several months after the study period as a peer-support group. This suggests some potential benefits for a sequential approach to transitioning from a professionally led to peer-led intervention, consistent with the CST study described above.

While many of the studies we reviewed above are based on peer support interventions developed for research studies but not currently widely available in communities, one study examined the experiences of individuals making use of a widely available peer support resource – peer support group meetings of the Depression and Bipolar Support Alliance (DBSA; formerly the National Depressive and Manic-Depressive Association). DBSA is a leading mental health consumer group serving the United States and Canada. DBSA provides group facilitators with opportunities for training in group leadership and up-to-date information about depression, and all groups have professional advisors (typically a psychiatrist, psychologist, nurse, or social worker) from the community. A survey of over 2000 individuals attending DBSA groups (DBSA, 2004) found that over 95% of respondents indicated that attending groups provided interpersonal support and helped them cope with problems and crises, as well as decision making. Over 85% indicated groups helped them understand medication and treatment, become more willing to take medication and cope with side effects and motivated to follow doctor's instructions, and become more effective at communicating with doctors. Longer attendance of DBSA groups was associated with fewer hospitalizations and lesser likelihood of stopping medications against doctor's instructions. Half of those who were non-adherent to their treatment plans became more adherent during the time they participated in the group. The non-randomized, naturalistic design of this study is likely positively biased to reflect the experiences of those who are most satisfied with DBSA groups. Nonetheless, these results suggest that benefits of peer support groups have the potential to generalize beyond controlled research studies.

Studies of individual peer support

One-on-one peer support programs have also received some research support. One such study targeted women who were at high risk for post-partum depression (Dennis, 2003) and were randomized to a telephone-based peer support program plus standard care or standard care alone (control group). Peer volunteers were women with a history of post-partum depression who attended a 4-hour training session focusing on telephone support and referral skills. Contact frequency was not standardized; on average, volunteers completed five 30-minute calls during the 2-month study period. The group that received peer support showed greater improvement in depression symptoms than the control group at 1-month and 2-month assessments.

One study tested a "befriending" intervention in which community volunteers were recruited to serve as peer supports to women with chronic depression living in inner city London identified by mail survey (Harris et al., 1999). Following 3 full days of training, volunteers met and talked with a depressed woman for at least 1 hour per week by "acting as a 'friend' to her, listening, and 'being there' for her." In addition to confiding, volunteers were encouraged to help befriendees to broaden their range of activities and offer practical support with ongoing difficulties. Depressed women were randomly assigned to the "befriending" or control condition. At a 1-year follow-up, 65% of the group allocated to befriending achieved remission, compared with only 39% of the control group.

A similar approach was employed in a recent open-trial pilot study of a peer-counseling program for elderly individuals with depression in Hong Kong (Ho, 2007). Although not a randomized controlled trial, this study is noteworthy for the model of professional and paraprofessional collaboration. The peer counselors were housewives and retirees who were recruited, screened, and trained by a psychiatric nurse and a social worker in a 13-hour, 6-week training course and practicum experience. Bimonthly meetings with peer counselors and trainers were held to provide support, and ongoing training was available upon request. Peer counselors were matched based on shared dialect, interests, and gender and interacted with the patients through monthly visits and weekly phone calls. Peer counselors submitted home visitation reports to trainers, which resulted in referral to the psychiatric nurse for re-assessment in cases of worsening symptoms. After participation in the program, depression symptoms decreased, and perceived health status, social support, and adaptive coping increased significantly.

In two of these studies (Dennis, 2003; Ho, 2007), peer volunteers were surveyed about their experience. The majority of peer volunteers indicated that participating contributed to their personal development. However, many reported times when they felt disappointed with the services they provided (Dennis, 2003) and with the extent of their training (Ho, 2007). Importantly, in both studies, peer supporters were instrumental in facilitating referrals to professional services.

Internet-based peer support interventions

Internet-based support groups are emerging as a promising new approach to gaining participation. As this is a newer area, controlled studies are limited. However, naturalistic studies support some of the hypothesized benefits of such groups in terms of reaching an underserved population. For instance, one observational study (Salem et al., 1997) analyzing the content of postings in several Internet-based depression support groups over a 2-week period found high usage rates by males, a group that is typically less likely to pursue conventional treatment for depression. Interestingly, the types of communications made by males and females were not significantly different. This suggests that the relative anonymity of Internet-based support groups may facilitate personal disclosure for males.

In a later study published in the *American Journal of Psychiatry* (Houston et al., 2002), researchers surveyed users of several existing web-based support groups and conducted a follow-up survey 1 year later. Consistent with the underserved population hypothesis, the sample tended to reflect an especially socially isolated group of patients with high chronicity and severity. Only a third ever attended a face-to-face support group meeting. In general, participants were highly satisfied with their experiences with the group, and nearly one third indicated that they would prefer an Internet-based support group to face-to-face counseling. Some but not all analyses suggest that high users (5 or more hours) were more likely to experience resolution of their depression symptoms than less frequent users. Given that this is a naturalistic study, one cannot conclude that group participation caused this improvement.

It is important to note that the researchers found little evidence to support the concern that participation in web-based groups would undermine professionally delivered treatment. In fact, most had discussed the support group with their provider, and many felt that it resulted in their being more active in their treatment. This finding is consistent with the proposed role of peer support groups in self-management. Taken together, the authors suggest that Internet-based support groups were promising; however, efforts to provide training to the individuals leading these groups would likely enhance their efficacy.

Although primarily a study of the efficacy of a computerized cognitive behavioral therapy (CBT) program, one study (Andersson et al., 2005) using an Internet-based discussion group as a control condition offers some insights on how to increase the utility of such discussion programs. In this study, participants with mild to moderate depression were assigned to either (1) a computerized CBT program and participation in an Internet-based discussion group with other program users, or (2) a discussion group only with other participants not receiving the CBT program. Not surprisingly, the combined treatment produced greater improvement than the discussion group alone. Participation in the discussion group alone tended to result in little benefit. Interestingly, the control group made nearly twice as many postings to their discussion group as the combined group; however, their postings tended to focus on personal problems and symptoms, whereas the combined group postings tended to focus on aspects of the CBT program. Taken together, these results raise some question about the utility of discussion groups outside the context of structured self-help.

Summary

Across the different peer support interventions, some trends emerged, suggesting what may lead to an optimal peer support interventions. More specifically, results suggest that overall, paraprofessionals can effectively deliver peer support interventions, with training typically lasting a few days. However, a structured intervention like CBT may be more effective in the hands of professional therapists (Bright et al., 1999). Moving beyond the question of relative efficacy of paraprofessionals versus professionals, two studies offered models of how peer leaders can facilitate referrals to professionals (Dennis, 2003; Ho, 2007). Indeed, the question of how to enhance collaboration between peer leaders and professionals is an important issue for further consideration. One way of fostering this relationship is through professionals providing supervision to peer leaders. Some studies made use of ongoing training and supervision of peer leaders (Bright et al., 1999; Ludman et al., 2007; Ho, 2007). As noted above, national organizations such as DBSA provide training programs for peer leaders. However, formal training may be less common in peer-initiated online support groups (Houston et al., 2002), and it is not clear how to facilitate such efforts.

It appears that the content of interventions may also be a crucial variable. One study found that a generic course on coping with chronic disease was less salient to some members than a program that provided information about coping specifically with depression (Ludman et al., 2007). It is also possible that integrating formal self-help materials into group meetings may allow a common text and set of strategies to facilitate more productive discussions (Andersson et al., 2005). Another way to accomplish this would be to form groups initially around a professionally delivered intervention and then encourage the group to transition into a peer support format (Ludman et al., 2007).

Limitations and challenges in peer support intervention research

As noted in the introduction, research on peer support groups typically is plagued by methodological flaws that limit definitive statements about its efficacy. To be fair, one clear challenge is that use of randomized controlled designs is not always feasible in studying naturally occurring peer support groups. We reviewed two relatively large longitudinal studies that found that regular participants in both face-to-face (DBSA, 2004) and Internet-based support groups (Houston et al., 2002) for depression show several improvements, including reduced depression symptoms and hospitalization and increased medication adherence. Although in both studies participants reported that the support group had been helpful, it is important to note that these are studies of self-selected individuals and as such may reflect more motivated or engaged patients. As such, without a control group, it is not possible to know if these individuals would have experienced similar improvements with the passage of time.

A newer generation of studies improves upon naturalistic studies by use of randomized designs as well as standardized training for individuals providing peer support. We reviewed several recent studies that make use of randomized designs; some (Dennis, 2003; Harris et al., 1999) but not all (den Boer et al., 2006; Ludman et al., 2007) find that peer support interventions were more effective in reducing depression symptoms than standard care. Some studies with negative findings may have lacked sufficient power to detect small differences or included control groups in which participants may have received unusually high-quality services. Also, some studies raise questions about the acceptability of peer support interventions to patients. Only half of the women approached for the befriending intervention expressed interest in receiving this service (Harris et al., 1999). In the study of cognitive self-therapy (CST; den Boer et al., 2006), slightly less than half of enrolled patients completed the CST initial skills course, and less than a third attended at least one self-therapy meeting, suggesting that it is the minority of patients who are willing to learn the presented skills and then provide this service to other patients in an ongoing manner. Finally, members of a peer-led disease management group were found to be less likely to attend follow-up sessions relative to members of the professionally led CBT group (Ludman et al., 2007). On balance, it is important to note that each of these limitations of the group interventions studied contributes clues that may lead to methods for improving the attractiveness of peer support interventions overall.

Finally, it is important to note that several of the reviewed studies published within the last 5 years were characterized by the authors as "pilot studies" (Dennis, 2003; Ho, 2007; Ludman et al., 2007). Although the small sample sizes in these studies present statistical limitations, this is a promising sign that more treatment development researchers are investigating strategies for optimizing the use of peer support in the treatment of depression. Similarly, the relative newness of Internet-based peer support programs suggests that high-quality studies of their efficacy will likely emerge in the coming years. Some have noted potential concern with Internet-based support groups, including potential for misinformation or hoaxes, verbal aggression or "flaming," withdrawal from non-Internet forms of social support, encouragement of suicide, and privacy issues (Eysenbach et al., 2004; Finfgeld, 2000; Lamberg, 2003). Although no such systematic problems have been reported in published reports (Eysenbach et al., 2004), it is likely that high-functioning groups are able to successful self-correct misinformation and limit participation from individuals who engage in disruptive or destructive behavior.

Practical issues

To whom to recommend peer support?

There is little formal evidence regarding what types of individuals are best suited to peer support interventions. Some data from the study of paraprofessional-versus professional-delivered CBT groups and mutual support groups described earlier (Bright et al., 1999) offer one possible clue. This study (Baker & Neimeyer, 2003) found that clients with a more "externalizing" style – those who view their problems in more situational terms – tended to benefit more from paraprofessional-delivered interventions; in contrast, individuals with a more "internalizing" style – those who tend to view their problems in more internal and psychological terms – tended to benefit more from professionally delivered interventions. The authors suggest that externalizing clients may respond best to the more common-sense and concrete suggestions made by paraprofessionals, whereas internalizing clients may view these responses as overly simplistic. However, given that these results emerged in the context of paraprofessionals delivering manualized interventions and this result has not yet been replicated, it would be premature to rule out peer support interventions for more internalizing clients.

In the absence of empirical data, some practical matters may inform which patients stand to gain the most from peer support interventions. The most obvious candidates would be individuals who lack social support. Some of the self-management strategies described in other chapters, such as exercise and bibliotherapy, appeared to be best suited to patients who are self-motivated and have developed some degree of self-efficacy. In contrast, peer support groups may not necessarily require the same degree of initiative outside of regular attendance. As described earlier, through contact with group leaders who have learned to successfully manage depression, group members may enhance their self-efficacy to initiate other self-management interventions. In the following section, we also consider how patient factors may guide the selection of the type of groups to recommend.

Role of clinician

Before a clinician considers recommending a peer support group, it is crucial that they examine their own attitudes towards peer support. There is evidence that some clinicians harbor suspicions about non-professionally delivered interventions (Norcross, 2006; Sheffield, 2003). A survey of over 1000 mental health professionals found that they routinely viewed peer-led groups less favorably than professionally led groups (Salzer et al., 1999). This reticence may translate to delayed referrals to peer support in their community. Indeed, 57% of mood disorder patients had been diagnosed for over a year before learning about peer support groups in their area (NDMA, 1999, cited in Sheffield, 2003). A survey of psychiatrists found that while just over three fourths of the sample referred patients with mood disorders to self-help groups and felt knowledgeable about them, only a third talked with their patients about self-help interventions (Powell et al, 2000b). Psychiatrists who held more positive beliefs about self-help groups (i.e. felt patients can obtain useful information and support) and less negative beliefs about self-help groups (i.e. felt groups were inappropriate and were concerned about lack of professional oversight) were more active proponents of self-help (e.g. made referrals to self-help groups, had literature from self-help groups on hand, and were professional affiliates of these groups). Interestingly, one of the strongest predictors of being an active proponent of self-help was having received education or information about self-help groups in the past 2 years. Although a causal link cannot be made from these results, it suggests that better-informed clinicians may hold groups in a more favorable light and make more active use of them for referrals. For instance, concern about lack of professional oversight may be reduced when psychiatrists learn more about the different ways peer support groups like DBSA and National Association of Mental Illness (NAMI) maintain contact with professionals. Also, by inviting discussion about patients' experiences in self-help groups, it is possible that any potentially inaccurate information could be countered.

How can clinicians become better educated about peer support groups? In Appendix A, we include websites for several national organizations with local meetings throughout the country. By visiting these websites, clinicians can learn about the types of training that peer leaders undergo. Sheffield (2003) also recommends several strategies for learning more about local peer support groups. An obvious strategy would be to attend a group meeting; however, not all self-help groups allow professionals to attend meetings as policy. For groups that do not allow clinicians to attend meetings, you may learn more about the group by speaking with the group leader on the telephone or volunteering to give a presentation on a professional topic to the group. In such contact, it would be important to inquire about areas of concern, such as how information about medication or other forms of treatment are handled. Another way to gain information would be to informally survey patients about their experiences in peer support groups in the area.

Once the clinician is well informed about the groups in their area, he/she may begin making referrals with confidence. As noted above, it is valuable to continue to inquire about the patient's group experiences as a means of supporting attendance and addressing any concerns that the patient has about information exchanged in the group.

What to recommend

Our first recommendation concerns peer support groups that are affiliated with national groups such as DBSA and NAMI. In Appendix A, we supply information on how to find local chapters of these organizations. Nonetheless, there is no guarantee that a local chapter at any given time will be of high quality or vitality. Also, patients may choose to seek out other types of group, for instance, informal groups that communicate through the Internet. To help patients evaluate groups, we developed Appendix B, which presents a list of favorable qualities and potential warning signs about peer support groups to help patients choose one that is likely to be rewarding.

Some patients may be reluctant to attend a peer support meeting due to potential misperceptions. One fear patients may have is that they will leave feeling more depressed due to members discussing their life circumstances in overly negative and unproductive terms. Although members will discuss challenges in their lives and even feelings of hopelessness, effective support groups encourage members to shift to more productive discussions of how to cope with problems. As Sheffield (2003) describes meetings she has observed: "It is an eye-opener to encounter little melodrama and self-pity and much practicality, determination, and humor" (p 90). For this reason, it may be helpful to encourage participants to attend a few meetings on a trial basis before making any longer-term commitments. It may also be helpful to encourage members to try more than one group to find one that is a good fit for their expectations (Powell et al., 2000b).

Another approach which may facilitate attendance is to arrange for a patient to have contact with a veteran member of a support group prior to attending their first meeting. One study found that mood disorder patients randomly assigned to receive such prior contact were more likely to later attend one or more meetings on their own relative to patients who had not received prior contact (Powell et al., 2000a). As such, it may be worth contacting the leader of a local chapter to learn if any members would be interested in providing such contact.

Some patients may feel uncomfortable attending a peer support group out of a concern with "burdening" other people with their problems. For such patients, it might be helpful to remind them that individuals who benefit most from peer support groups are those who give support as well as receive it (e.g. Maton, 1988).

Another decision is whether to recommend an online support group or a face-to-face group. As noted above, there is no reason the patient could not try both. Each offers unique benefits. Participation in a face-to-face meeting offers the benefits of engaging with a local community. As such, it is possible for patients to exchange information about resources in the regions as well as potential recommendations for clinicians (Sheffield, 2003). For socially isolated patients, it may provide a useful behavioral activation assignment to attend a group. Other opportunities for reinforcing activities and outside group friendships may also be more likely to follow from this format.

Several specific benefits of online groups have been described (Finfgeld, 2000; Lamberg, 2003). Some may prefer the anonymity of an online support group due to social anxiety or fear of loss of confidentiality. While some online support groups have regularly scheduled meeting times, many offer opportunities to participate around the clock by reading and replying to postings or chatting with someone in real time. For patients in more remote areas or with limited transportation or physical disabilities, online support groups may be the most viable option. Online support programs also offer the opportunity to "lurk," or read messages and observe group dynamics, so a person will feel more comfortable participating.

A final question is what type of group would make an appropriate referral. Some support groups are specific to depression or mood disorders. These may be particularly helpful for individuals for whom better understanding and accep-tance of this diagnosis would be helpful (e.g. DBSA). Other groups address a broader range of mental illness (e.g. NAMI) and may be appropriate for individ-uals with significant comorbidity with anxiety or psychotic disorders. For indi-viduals whose depression is clearly linked to a specific stressor (e.g. parenting, care giving, specific medical conditions, retirement), finding a group focused on these concerns may be more relevant than one focused solely on mood disorders. A clearing house for support groups for a range of medical, psychiatric, and life-adjustment concerns is located at http://www.mentalhelp.net/selfhelp/.

A final type of group may be appropriate for patients who "over-identify" with the diagnostic label. As such, it might be useful to encourage participation in activities that help to reinforce other aspects of the individual's self-concept (e.g. religious, community service, political activism, athletic, or other recreational organization). Although this strategy has not been formally evaluated as an intervention for depression, encouraging patients to engage in environments that offer potential for positive reinforcement and development of mastery would be consistent with the behavioral activation component of cognitive behavioral therapy (CBT).

Additional self-management approaches for enhancing social support

The primary focus of this chapter is on peer support groups due to their widespread availability in the community. However, a recent review of interventions designed to increase social support concludes that such peer groups may not be entirely sufficient to address social support needs (Hogan et al., 2002). The authors recommend also finding ways to involve members of the individual's naturally occurring support network, namely family members and friends. In addition, some patients may benefit from guidance by group members on how to build support outside of groups, for instance, through social skills training. Interestingly, this recommendation came from reviewing social support interventions designed for a range of disorders; however, it is especially relevant for depression, which is increasingly being understood not merely as the result of low social support, but instead in terms of a complex interplay of interpersonal factors (Joiner & Coyne, 1999) involving both the person with depression and those in his/her social network (i.e. family and friends). We highlight some of these basic research findings and discuss ways that these factors may be ameliorated through interventions directed to family and friends and to the patient themselves.

Involving family and friends

Family and friends may be the first to recognize symptoms (Highnet et al., 2005). However, they may not fully understand what exactly is happening and how to respond most effectively. When well-meaning attempts to make a person feel better do not result in improvement, a loved one may begin to feel discouraged and helpless (Coyne, 1976). Alternatively, when helping efforts do not lead to improvement, family members may also feel frustrated or resentful and begin communicating towards the depressed individual in a manner that is excessively critical and hostile. Research studies have shown that such a communication style is very likely to worsen the individual's depression symptoms (Butzlaff & Hooley, 1998). As such, it is crucial that family members and friends not be neglected in the self-management process.

Given that members of the general public may not be knowledgeable of the best way to respond when a loved one is depressed, a recent study (Langlands et al., 2008) was conducted in which a group of 167 mental health consumers (i.e. individuals with a history of depression), caregivers, and clinicians from several English-speaking countries were surveyed with the goal of developing a consensus statement on effective "first-aid" strategies for depression. Statements endorsed by 80% or more of the panelists were retained. We have summarized this consensus statement in a hand-out that can be given to friends or family members who are concerned about someone with depression (see Appendix C). These strategies provide concrete guidelines for how to provide support and encourage the uptake of appropriate professional help.

Family members and friends are also encouraged to seek out accurate and reliable information about depression. This can be accomplished in several ways. First, the clinician can direct them to any one of the informational websites listed in Table 4.1 in the Self-Help chapter. Second, several national organizations offer informational sessions and support groups for the family members of individuals with depression and other mental illnesses. For instance, the National Alliance for the Mentally Ill offers 12-week courses to educate family members about depression and other major psychiatric disorders. The Depression and Bipolar Support Alliance offers community and Internet-based support groups for family members of individuals with mood disorders. Internet addresses for both organizations are listed in Table 4.1.

Steps a patient can take to increase their social support

As described in the beginning of this chapter, individuals with depression often lack adequate social support and tend to be dissatisfied with the support they have. The previous two sections have explored strategies to increase available support for patients through peer support groups and mobilizing family members and friends. However, as described earlier, there is considerable evidence that individuals with depression may engage in several interpersonal habits that may erode available social support. Informed by their own research on interpersonal processes in depression as well as over 30 years of work by their colleagues, Pettit and Joiner (2005) developed a self-help book that seeks to increase the awareness of individuals with depression about counterproductive interpersonal habits as well as strategies for shifting into more productive habits. This book is entitled *The Interpersonal Solution to Depression: A Workbook for Changing How You Feel by Changing How You Relate.* Counterproductive habits addressed in this book include depressive communication styles, devaluing the social skills they do have, interpersonal avoidance, disclosing personal shortcomings, self-sabotage, soliciting negative feedback, and excessively seeking reassurance. Appendix D describes these habits in more detail and includes information for patients on the self-help book that contains strategies for addressing these patterns.

This is not to say that all patients with depression have social skills deficits. However, clinicians may get a sense that some patients would be good candidates for this type of intervention based on the patients' description of interpersonal problems or the clinicians' own impressions based on first-hand interactions. However, it is important to introduce this recommendation in a thoughtful and sensitive manner. When a clinician states that a patient lacks social skills, this may have several unintended negative consequences. For example, this may be heard as criticism and potentially provoke a defensive reaction such as refusing to explore this intervention. This may also feed into a patient's already low sense of self. Finally, the mere suggestion that a patient may be engaging in some behavior that contributes to one's depression may lead some patients to feel that they are being "blamed as the victim."

To avoid such misunderstandings, we recommend introducing this topic in a non-confrontational manner and framing the discussion as an opportunity to develop coping skills consistent with other self-management strategies. For instance, the topic may be introduced by asking whether they feel as though their interactions with people have not been going as well as they have at other times when they were not feeling depressed. If the person agrees, the clinician can normalize this by acknowledging that this happens to many people with depression and that researchers have identified several counterproductive interpersonal habits that may contribute to depression. The clinician can then ask the patient if he or she would be interested in reading more about these habits and – if any seem relevant to their own situation – learning some strategies for shifting into more effective habits. If the patient expresses interest, clinicians can provide them with Appendix D, which includes a summary of these ineffective interpersonal habits and a reference to Pettit's and Joiner's (2005) self-help guide that includes exercises for changing these habits. We should note that unlike other bibliotherapy resources described in this book, the efficacy of this book has not been tested in a controlled study. However, it is based on a well-researched model of depression, makes use of specific activities, provides reasonable expectations about the types of gains possible, and contains information on preventing relapse. As such, it is consistent with recently presented guidelines for determining the quality and utility of a mental health self-help book (Redding et al., in press).

It is important to recognize that the self-management strategies described above are designed to complement traditional treatment. It is important to recognize that, for some patients, interpersonal factors may need to be a focus of professional interventions. Several psychotherapies that focus explicitly on interpersonal aspects of depression have received considerable empirical support. These include interpersonal psychotherapy (IPT; Klerman et al., 1984; Weissman & Markowitz, 2002), behaviorally oriented marital therapy (Jacobson et al., 1991; O'Leary & Beach, 1990), and cognitive behavioral analysis system of psychotherapy (CBASP; McCullough, 2000). Including appropriate attention to interpersonal factors in professional interventions will likely enhance the utility of the self-management strategies described above.

Summary and conclusions

Peer support interventions are a valuable component of self-management for depression in that they can augment the traditional clinician–patient relationship, be a source of information, promote self-monitoring and treatment adherence, and increase a patient's self-efficacy for coping with depression. The emerging body of research suggests that peers and other non-professionals can effectively deliver supportive interventions with minimal training and supervision. The small body of controlled research trials also suggests that peer support interventions show promise in depression symptoms, whereas non-controlled observational studies point to additional benefits such as increased medication adherence and reduced hospitalization. Clinicians can play a valuable role in introducing patients to peer support groups in the community. In addition to promoting peer support groups, clinicians may also wish to consider interventions to enhance the patient's naturally occurring sources of support. As such, we discussed strategies to help family members and friends provide effective support to a person with depression and provide information to patients about interpersonal behavior that may undermine potentially supportive relationships.

REFERENCES

Brown GW, Harris TO. *Social Origins of Depression: A Study of Psychiatric Disorders in Women.* London: Tavistock; 1978.

Andersson G, Bergstrom J, Hollandare F, Carlbring P, Kaldo V, Ekselius L. Internet-based self-help for depression: randomized controlled trial. *Br J Psychiatry.* 2005; 187:456–461.

Baker KD, Neimeyer RA. Therapist training and client characteristics as predictors of treatment response to group therapy for depression. *Psychother Res.* 2003; 13(2):135–151.

Bandura A. *Self-Efficacy: The Exercise of Control.* New York, NY: W.H. Freeman; 1997.

Bright JI, Baker KD, Neimeyer RA. Professional and paraprofessional group treatments for depression: a comparison of cognitive-behavioral and mutual support interventions. *J Consult Clin Psychol.* 1999; 67(4):491–501.

Butzlaff RL, Hooley JM. Expressed emotion and psychiatric relapse. *Arch Gen Psychiatry.* 1998; 55:547–552.

Coyne JC. Toward an interactional description of depression. *Psychiatry.* 1976; 39(1): 28–40.

Davison KP, Pennebaker JW, Dickerson SS. Who talks? The social psychology of illness support groups. *Am Psychol.* 2000; 55:205–217.

Depression and Bipolar Support Alliance. *DBSA Support Groups: A Important Step on the Road to Wellness.* Chicago, IL: DBSA; 2004. Brochure.

den Boer PCAM, Wiersma D, van Den Bosch RJ. Paraprofessionals for anxiety and depressive disorders. *Cochrane Database Syst Rev.* 2005; (2):CD004688.

den Boer PCAM, Wiersma D, Vaarwerk IT, Span MM, Stant AD, van Den Bosch RJ. Cognitive self-therapy for chronic depression and anxiety: a multi-centre randomized controlled study. *Psychol Med.* 2006; 1–11.

Dennis CL. The effect of peer support on postpartum depression: a pilot randomized controlled trial. *Can J Psychiatry.* 2003; 48(2):115–124.

Eysenbach G, Powell J, Englesakis M, Rizo C, Stern A. Health related virtual communities and electronic support groups: systematic review of the effects of online peer to peer interactions. *Br Med J.* 2004; 328:1–6.

Finfgeld DL. Therapeutic groups online: the good, the bad, and the unknown. *Issues Ment Health Nurs.* 2000; 21:241–255.

Harris T, Brown GW, Robinson R. Befriending as an intervention for chronic depression among women in an inner city. *Br J Psychiatry.* 1999; 174:219–224.

Highnet N, Thompson M, McNair B. Identifying depression in a family member: the carers' experience. *J Affect Disorder.* 2005; 87:25–33.

Ho APY. A peer counseling program for the elderly with depression living in the community. *Aging Ment Health.* 2007; 11(1):69–74.

Hogan BE, Linden W, Najarian B. Social support interventions: do they work? *Clin Psychol Rev.* 2002; 22:381–440.

Houston TK, Cooper LA, Ford DE. Internet support groups for depression: a 1-year prospective cohort study. *Am J Psychiatry.* 2002; 159(12):2062– 2068.

Jacobson NS, Dobson KS, Fruzzetti A, Schmaling KB, Salusky S. Social-learning based marital therapy as a treatment for depression. *J Consult Clin Psychol.* 1991; 59:547–553.

Joiner TE Jr. Shyness and low social support as interactive diathesis, with loneliness as a mediator: testing an interpersonal-personality view of vulnerability to depression. *J Abnorm Psychol.* 1997; 106(3):386–394.

Joiner TE Jr, Coyne JC. *Interactional Nature of Depression: Advances in Interpersonal Approaches.* Washington, DC: American Psychological Association; 1999.

Kendler KS, Myers J, Prescott CA. Sex differences in the relationship between the relationship between social support and the risk for major depression: a longitudinal study of opposite-sex twin pairs. *Am J Psychiatry.* 2005; 162:250–256.

Kessler RC, Mickelson KD, Zhao S. Patterns and correlates of self-help group membership in the United States. *Soc Policy.* 1997; 27:27–46.

Klerman GL, Weissman M, Rounsaville BJ, Chevron ES. *Interpersonal Therapy for Depression.* New York, NY: Basic Books; 1984.

Lamberg L. Online empathy for mood disorders: patients turn to internet support groups. *J Am Med Assoc.* 2003; 289(23):3073–3077.

Langlands RL, Jorm AF, Kelly CM, Kitchener BA. First aid for depression: a Delphi consensus study with consumers, carers, and clinicians. *J Affect Disord*. 2008; 105:157–165.

Ludman EJ, Simon GE, Grothaus LC, Luce C, Markley DK, Schaefer J. A pilot study of telephone care management and structured disease self-management groups for chronic depression. *Psychiatr Serv*. 2007; 58(8):1065–1072.

Maton KI. Social support, organizational characteristics, psychological well-being, and group appraisal in three self-help group populations. *Am J Commun Psychol*. 1988; 16:53–77.

McCullough JP. *Treatment for Chronic Depression: Cognitive Behavioral Analysis System of Psychotherapy*. New York, NY: Guilford Press; 2000.

Norcross JC. Integrating self-help into psychotherapy: 16 practical suggestions. *Prof Psychol Res Pract*. 2006; 37(6):683–693.

O'Leary KD, Beach SRH. Marital therapy: a viable treatment for depression and marital discord. *Am J Psychiatry*. 1990; 147:183–186.

Pettit JW, Joiner TE. *The Interpersonal Solution to Depression: A Workbook for Changing How You Feel by Changing How You Relate*. Oakland, CA: New Harbinger Publications; 2005.

Powell TJ, Hill EM, Warner L, Yeaton W, Silk K. Encouraging people with mood disorders to attend a self-help group. *J Appl Soc Psychol*. 2000a; 30:2270–2288.

Powell TJ, Silk KR, Albeck J. Psychiatrists' referrals to self-help groups for people with mood disorders. *Psychiatr Serv*. 2000b; 51:809–811.

Redding RE, Herbert JD, Forman EM, Gaudiano BA. Popular self-help books for anxiety, depression, and trauma: how scientifically grounded and useful are they? *Prof Psychol Res Pr* 2008; 39:537–545.

Salem DA, Bogat GA, Reid C. Mutual help goes on-line. *J Commun Psychol*. 1997; 25(2):189–207.

Salzer MS, Rappaport J, Segre L. Professional appraisal of professionally led and self-help groups. *Am J Orthopsychiatry*. 1999; 69(4):536–540.

Seligman MEP. The effectiveness of psychotherapy. *Am Psychol*. 1995; 50:965–974.

Sheffield A. Referral to a peer-led support group: An effective aid for mood disorder patients. *Prim Psychiatry*. 2003; 10(5):89–94.

Sherbourne CD, Hays RD, Wells KB. Personal and psychosocial risk factors for physical and mental health outcomes and course of depression among depressed patients. *J Consult Clin Psychol*. 1995; 63(3):345–355.

Wagner EH. Chronic disease management: what will it take to improve care for chronic illness. *Effect Clin Pract*. 1998; 1:2–4.

Weissman MM, Markowitz JC. Interpersonal psychotherapy for depression. In Gotlib IH and Hammen CL, eds. *Handbook of Depression*. New York, NY: Guilford Press; 2002, pp 404–421.

Appendix A   Tips for finding a peer support group

Peer support groups exist to provide members with the opportunity to give and receive emotional support and to exchange information and encouragement. The peers who provide the support are typically individuals who have first-hand experience with depression. Peer support groups have traditionally involved face-to-face meetings but are increasingly available through the Internet. Below is a list of national organizations that offer peer support resources across the United States in the form of face-to-face meetings in local communities and Internet-based communities.

Organization	Web address	Focus of group	Community groups meetings	Alternative to group meetings
Depression and Bipolar Support Alliance (DBSA)	www.dbsalliance.org	Mood disorders	Yes; US and Canada	Many Internet-based discussion groups as well as virtual support group meetings for both mental health consumers and family members
National Alliance for the Mentally Ill	www.nami.org	Mood and anxiety disorders, schizophrenia	Yes; US including DC and Puerto Rico	Internet-based discussion groups
Depression and Related Affective Disorders Association (DRADA)	www.drada.org	Mood disorders	Yes, largely in Mid-Atlantic region of the US	Peer support program matches individuals with depression and family members who wish to email, write or talk with others with similar concerns.
Walkers in Darkness, Inc.	www.walkers.org	Mood disorders	No	Internet-based discussion groups and chat room features

Another valuable resource for identifying community and Internet-based support groups is the American Self-Help Clearinghouse (http://www.mentalhelp.net/selfhelp/). This organization provides listings of support groups for a range of medical, psychiatric, and life adjustment issues. This may be a helpful place to look for groups that address issues other than depression or that present alternative support group formats for addressing depression and other mental health issues. It also provides links to self-help and mutual support groups in countries other than the United States.

Appendix B   Tips for selecting a peer support group

Exchanging information, support, and encouragement with other people with first-hand experience coping with depression is a unique and valuable complement to traditional forms of treatment such as medication and psychotherapy. By definition, peer support groups are typically not led by medical or mental health professionals. In many but certainly not all cases, group facilitators receive some training in leading a group from national organizations. However, just as there is variability in the quality of trained medical and mental health professionals, there is also variability in terms of the quality of support groups. For this reason, it can be difficult to know for sure how effective any given peer support group will be for you before trying it out. If you have never attended a

What to expect	Warning signs
Group leaders, members, and visiting experts provide scientifically based information on depression and its treatment	Inaccurate theories about causes of depression and untested treatments for depression are promoted or presented without critical discussion
Members listen to discussions of hardship, offer support and encouragement, and facilitate active problem solving where appropriate.	Members allow one another to complain or indulge in self-pity without encouraging members to take responsibility for coping when possible.
Members maintain a positive and optimistic tone and sense of humor.	Tone of meeting is dominated by cynical or discouraging comments.
When a member discusses frustrations with treatment such as side effects, slow rate of improvement, and feeling misunderstood by their clinician, group members encourage adherence with prescribed treatment and discuss constructive solutions such as strategies for effective clinician–patient communication and seeking a second opinion.	Members engage in "doctor-bashing" or recommend stopping a treatment. Group members pressure members to discontinue medication or other forms of professionally delivered treatment without first consulting their clinician. Group members aggressively market a product (for example, herbal remedies or personal enhancement programs).
Group members offer constructive ideas about increasing social support and solving interpersonal challenges presented by depression	Group members discourage participation in relationships with people not part of the support group.
Members values the safety of other members	Although rare, "extreme groups" on the Internet that support suicide have been documented and should be avoided.

peer support group meeting, you may be reluctant to try one because you don't know what to expect. Alternatively, you may have had an unpleasant experience with a group you tried in the past. For this reason, we have assembled a list of qualities that it is reasonable to expect in an effective peer support group. We have also included a list of warning signs that may characterize less effective groups and may serve as warning signs that it is useful to try a different peer support group.

Appendix C   How can family and friends help when a loved one is depressed?

Family members and friends are often the first to notice when a loved one is developing depression and provide daily support. Even though you may feel concerned, you may not feel confident in knowing how to be supportive and when to recommend that a person receive help. Below are some suggestions based on the recommendations drawn from a recent survey of health care providers, individuals who have experienced depression, and friends and family members who have cared for someone with depression. The citation for this study is listed at the end of this hand-out.

Recognize and understand the symptoms of depression

- Know the symptoms of depression (sad or irritable mood; loss of interest in previously enjoyed activities; changes in appetite and sleep; loss of energy; agitation; excessive self-criticism; changes in attention, memory, or concentration; thinking or talking about death or suicide).
- Inform yourself about the causes of and treatment for depression from a reliable source, such as the National Institute for Mental Health (http://www. nimh.nih.gov/health/topics/depression/index.shtml).
- Don't assume depression will go away on its own.

Approach the person with depression

- Communicate that you are concerned.
- Give the person reasonable opportunities to talk about how he or she has been feeling and what is on his or her mind. Ask how long he or she has been feeling this way.
- Select a time and location where you will both be comfortable talking. Remember: talking about depression won't make it worse. However, if the person does not feel comfortable talking, avoid pressuring him or her. Instead, make clear you are willing to listen when he or she is ready. You can also encourage him or her to talk with another trusted individual (e.g. friend, family member, clergy, or health care professional).
- Be sure to really listen. Be patient as the person may talk more slowly and be thinking less clearly than usual. Don't interrupt. It may help to try to summarize what the person has said to make sure you understand it before offering your opinion. If he or she says things that seem overly pessimistic or irrational, it may be helpful to gently offer a different perspective, but avoid arguing.

Offering help and being supportive

- Communicate that you are willing to help and that you will stick with them.
- Ask if the person would like information about depression and direct him or her to reliable information. However, don't assume the person doesn't already know about depression.
- Misunderstanding and negative attitudes towards depression are unfortunately all too common. A person with depression may have internalized these ideas or fear that you believe these things. Therefore, it is important to communicate the following:
  - Depression is a medical illness.
  - You don't blame the person or think less of him or her for experiencing depression.
  - You don't think depression is really a matter of character flaws such as being "weak," "lazy," "selfish," or "trying to get attention."
- Offer a reasonable amount of practical assistance with daily tasks that may feel overwhelming for the person with depression (e.g. cleaning the house, grocery shopping).
- Be understanding, compassionate, patient, and accepting of the person. Be prepared that your kindness and attention may not be reciprocated.
- Don't be overly worried about saying the wrong thing. It is better to err on the side of communicating caring. However, some forms of communication should certainly be avoided, including hostility, sarcasm, and trivializing of the depressed person's symptoms. Do not blame the person for feeling down. It will not help to tell a person to "get over it," "cheer up," or "look on the bright side."
- Convey hope that, with time and treatment, depression and the situations that contribute to it will improve, even if it doesn't seem like it right now.

Encouraging seeking treatment

- When symptoms of depression have persisted for several weeks, suggest that the person seek professional help to receive an accurate diagnosis and effective treatment.
- Discuss the options the person has for seeking help. Offer to help research options, for instance, by calling his or her insurance company.
- Offer to accompany him or her to an initial appointment, but allow space for the person to speak for him/herself and make his or her own decisions.
- If the person feels misunderstood or discouraged by the first health care provider consulted, encourage him/her to continue looking until he/she can find a provider with whom he or she can establish a good working relationship. The extra time and effort is worth it in the long run.

What if the person won't seek treatment?

- Try to clarify the reasons the person won't seek treatment. If this decision is based on mistaken beliefs, try to provide accurate information (for example, discuss perceived financial constraints, remind them that their privacy will be protected, effective treatments are available, and only in emergency situations would treatment involve hospitalization).
- You may also mention that some forms of self-help have been shown to help some individuals reduce their depression symptoms. For example, the book *Feeling Good* by David Burns, M.D., has been supported in several research studies. However, be sensitive that self-help may feel like an overwhelming undertaking for someone who is depressed.
- Let the person know that you are willing to help if he or she decides to pursue professional help at a later time.
- Respect his or her right to not seek help unless you believe the person is at risk of harming him or herself or others. In this circumstance, contact a medical professional on his or her behalf or bring them to the nearest emergency room.

Respect your own limits

- Resist the urge to try to cure the person yourself or solve all of his or her problems.
- Do not neglect your own self-care when providing support to someone with depression. Take time to engage in activities that provide relaxation and rejuvenation.
- Consider attending a support group for family members of people with depression and other psychological disorders. The Depression and Bipolar Support Alliance (www.dbsalliance.org) and the National Alliance for the Mentally Ill (www.nami.org) have resources to offer support and information for the families of individuals with depression and other mental health problems.

Source: Langlands RL, Jorm AF, Kelly CM, Kitchener BA. First aid for depression: a Delphi consensus study with consumers, carers, and clinicians.

*J Affect Disord.*2007; 105:157–165.

Appendix D   Six interpersonal habits that can make depression worse

Researchers have identified six counterproductive interpersonal habits that put people at risk for developing depression and keeping them stuck in depression by hurting their relationships, self-esteem, and chances of experiencing positive events. Below are brief descriptions of these habits.

Depressive communication: People with depression may tend to dwell on negative topics in conversation and make critical comments about themselves and others. They may also use verbal and non-verbal behavior that communicates a lack of confidence, such as speaking softly and avoiding eye contact.

Underestimating social skills: Individuals with depression tend to see themselves as less socially skilled than others see them. In other words, they may over-emphasize their less effective habits and minimize their effective ones.

Interpersonal avoidance: People with depression may be unassertive, avoid interpersonal conflict, and withdraw from social contact. These behaviors in turn produce disappointment, prevent problems from getting solved, and reduce opportunities for eventually experiencing positive outcomes – all of which maintain depression.

Selling oneself short: People with depression may disclose personal shortcomings more readily than non-depressed individuals. Individuals with depression may also engage in forms of self-sabotage to provide a ready-made excuse for things that don't go well (for example, failing to prepare for an important presentation).

Negative feedback seeking: People with depression may reject compliments from others and instead seek out negative comments from people because this is more consistent with how they feel about themselves. This can lead to interpersonal rejection, which in turn maintains depression.

Excessive reassurance seeking: In contrast to negative feedback seeking, people with depression may repeatedly ask others for confirmation that they are indeed worthwhile. This can also lead to interpersonal rejection, which in turn maintains depression.

If you catch yourself engaging in these patterns, you may wish to read *The Interpersonal Solution to Depression: A Workbook for Changing How You Feel by Changing How You Relate* by Jeremy W. Pettit, Ph.D., and Thomas E. Joiner, Jr., Ph.D., a self-help book which describes these patterns in more detail and provides practical strategies for how to shift into more productive interpersonal habits. You may also wish to discuss these patterns with the clinician who is providing your treatment for depression.

Source: Pettit JW, Joiner TE. *The Interpersonal Solution to Depression: A Workbook for Changing How You Feel by Changing How You Relate.* Oakland, CA: New Harbinger Publications; 2005.

Putting it all together

Applying self-management for depression in your practice

In the preceding chapters, we have presented a rationale for the integration of self-management into the treatment of depression in both primary care and mental health settings. We have discussed how self-management is promoted through a collaborative relationship between clinicians and patients and can be further strengthened by the use of care managers. We have also reviewed the research support for several components of self-management, including self-assessment, exercise, self-help psychotherapy programs, peer support groups, and meditation. We have also presented some practical recommendations for applying these approaches with your patients. This final chapter focuses on how to translate these findings and recommendations into concrete changes in your own clinical practice.

As we said in the outset of this book, self-management is not a one-size-fits-all approach. As clinicians working in the self-management model, we acknowledge the importance of matching clinicians' strategies with patients' goals in a collaborative manner. As authors, we wish to maintain this philosophy. In this book, one objective has been to present an overview of a range of self-management approaches. We believe that not all of these strategies will be equally useful to each clinician or equally relevant to each treatment setting. Self-management can address many of the challenges clinicians face in treating depression; however, the specific challenges differ from practice to practice. Also in keeping with our model of self-management, we acknowledge that behavioral change is effortful and does not automatically follow from the acquisition of new information. Indeed, in previous chapters, we discussed the barriers that may prevent patients from using self-management techniques.

In this final chapter, we first present a few common challenges faced in the delivery of depression treatment across various settings as a jumping-off point to review some of the ways that specific aspects of self-management may help improve practice effectiveness. We will also address some of the barriers that clinicians may face in implementing self-management strategies, as well as strategies for overcoming these challenges.

What challenges does your practice face and how can self-management help?

Depression is a complex and challenging problem to treat. Due to its complexity, it can be difficult to manage in settings where time with patients is limited. Furthermore, it can be frustrating to watch patients experience limited relief from conventional treatments and even more frustrating to watch patients relapse after successful treatments. In addition, not all patients have access to the resources needed to achieve optimal outcomes. Below, we address these and other challenges and describe how self-management strategies may be relevant.

Too little time with each patient

An increasing reality of the current model of managed care is that clinicians often do not have as much time as they may wish to spend with each patient. Some of the self-management approaches described in this book may help to address this challenge. For primary care clinicians, this may take the form of increasingly shorter appointments as physicians and nurse practitioners work to fit more patients into each day. In the course of assessing all other systems of health, it is not always possible to fully assess depression. Given that undetected depression can contribute to poorer health and functioning, depression screening with self-assessment tools before the visit may be a useful way of both detecting depression and highlighting symptoms that require further assessment during the visit. Furthermore, as the number of patients seen increases, follow-up with each patient can become increasingly difficult. As such, care managers can become a vital liaison between a patient and clinicians by providing education about depression, supervising behavioral interventions such as exercise plans, and answering questions about medication such as side effects. Monitoring changes in depressive symptoms following treatment with self-assessment tools before each follow-up visit in primary care can also facilitate caring for depressed patients.

In mental health care settings, this issue of having too little time with patients can take the form of challenges in obtaining authorization from the patient's insurance company for a sufficient number of sessions. You want to use every precious minute of each session on building therapeutic alliance, exploring the historical and current factors that maintain the patient's depression, developing a customized plan for coping and behavior change, and troubleshooting when coping efforts do not lead to desired outcomes. One strategy for making the most of each precious minute of each session is to use self-management resources for therapeutic tasks that do not require your expertise as a clinician to implement. For instance, having patients complete self-assessments and submit them to you at the beginning of each session can give you a comprehensive and up-to-date snapshot of a patient's depression symptom severity without sacrificing time in session to assessing all areas of symptoms. Referring patients to websites to obtain information about treatment can cut down on time spent educating the patient about the diagnosis. Self-help resources can help structuring home practice and reinforce aspects of treatment presented in session.

Patients do not experience sufficient improvement with treatment or experience frequent relapse

A frustrating reality is that not all patients respond adequately to first-line pharmacological and psychotherapy treatments. As such, some of the self-management strategies described in this book may be thought of as helpful complementary or augmentation strategies. For instance, we presented emerging evidence that exercise and meditation may be useful adjunctive self-administered treatments for patients who partially respond to pharmacological interventions.

Another factor in partial recovery is non-adherence to prescribed treatment. When patients do not adhere to prescribed treatments, it is a unilateral treatment decision on the part of the patient. The collaborative care approach helps to empower patients to make treatment decisions within the context of information and support from their provider. We presented evidence that peer support groups may also help foster treatment adherence. Group members can provide information, encouragement, and support with issues such as coping with medication side effects. They can also provide tips to help patients effectively communicate with providers.

The chronicity of depression is well known to clinicians and researchers alike. The self-management approach to depression described in this book is informed by models developed for the comprehensive treatment of other chronic disorders such as diabetes and obesity. The self-management perspective helps to involve the patient as an active partner in managing depression. By encouraging patients to self-monitor symptoms, clinicians will be able to better detect early relapse. By providing patients with tools for self-management such as exercise and coping skills introduced in self-help resources, patients will be better prepared to address prodromal symptoms. For instance, we presented evidence from multiple studies that mindfulness meditation can help prevent relapse among patients with chronic depression.

Patients in our setting have limited access to mental health care

Depending on a variety of factors, many patients have difficulty accessing mental health specialty care. As noted above, primary care clinicians often do not have the time or resources to treat depression beyond basic pharmacological interventions. Some geographic regions have limited options for referrals to psychiatrists, psychologists, or social workers. In other settings, long waitlists mean that patients' conditions may further deteriorate as they await their first appointment with a psychopharmacologist or psychotherapist. Other barriers to receiving mental health care include limited mobility and transportation, stigma, and lack of insurance benefits. In other cases, patients may simply not have the time to follow-up with additional appointments.

For each of these challenges, various self-management approaches may be useful. When referral options are limited, one strategy is to tap into other resources for mental health care outside of conventional treatment outlets. This may include a referral to a peer support group or an exercise program in the community. Self-help interventions may be a useful method of introducing empirically supported psychotherapy to patients on waitlists for mental health care. This stepped care approach may ultimately reduce the amount of sessions patients need once they eventually begin treatment with a mental health specialist. We presented evidence that psychoeducational self-help programs can help to reduce patients' sense of stigma associated with a diagnosis of depression, and self-help interventions can also provide an anonymous method for accessing help for those who continue to resist seeking mental health care. The increased use of Internet-based self-assessment, self-help, and peer support groups offers considerable promise for reaching patients who are unable to physically access mental health specialty care due to barriers of geography, mobility, transportation, or time.

Difficulty attracting patients to a private practice

As noted above, some clinicians may feel overwhelmed by the volume of patients with depression they are treating. However, some clinicians in private practice may face a different obstacle: maintaining a target caseload in competitive geographical regions. As we discussed in the chapter on self-help, some private practice clinicians may view self-management as a further threat to building their practice. However, the integration of self-management principles may help to distinguish your practice from others in the minds of potential clients and referral sources. Indeed, a hybrid practice blending conventional mental health interventions with self-management alternative and complementary approaches such as exercise or meditation may attract patients seeking a more holistic approach to wellness. A practice that integrates self-help program resources with professional consultation may attract highly motivated clients who might otherwise not seek psychotherapy. Work with such clients may be especially rewarding.

Depression is costing our organization too much

This section may be less relevant to individual clinicians and more to individuals whose professional roles cause them to think systemically about mental health care delivery. These can include individuals working in health maintenance organizations (HMOs), benefits managers in a workplace, or public policy makers – all of whom are well aware that treating depression with ongoing medication and psychotherapy can also be costly. We would argue that this is money well spent, when one considers the considerable costs associated with untreated or poorly managed depression, including disability, lost workplace productivity, and health care expenses for other conditions worsened by chronic depression. HMOs and workplaces are increasingly looking to self-management as a way to offer low-cost programs, such as computerized self-help programs. As we noted elsewhere in the book, evidence is accumulating that self-management may enhance the cost-effectiveness of depression treatment.

Overcoming barriers to implementing self-management

At this point, you may be persuaded that self-management could be helpful for the patients with depression that you see in your practice. After reading the section above, you may even have one or more specific components of self-management in mind that you feel is a strong match for addressing a specific challenge you face in your practice setting. However, as clinicians, we all know that knowledge alone does not necessarily lead to behavioral change. Clinicians wishing to implement changes in their practice can face very real barriers, including time pressures, as well as resistance from patients, colleagues, or the larger institution in which they work. In the following section, we discuss some of these challenges, along with incremental strategies for incorporating self-management into your practice.

Where will I find the time to make this change to my practice?

Many clinicians struggle to find the time to meet their existing commitments in the workplace associated with providing patient care – never mind taking on a major renovation to their practice. It is important to realize that integrating self-management into your practice can be done incrementally. Once you have identified the aspect of self-management that is most relevant to your practice, focus on the small but essential first steps. Often, these can be broken up into tasks that can fit into small windows of time during the day. For instance, you may begin by identifying and researching peer support groups in your community by visiting some of the websites listed in this book. You may seek out resources in your community where patients can join exercise programs or learn one of the forms of meditation described earlier. Discovering and reaching out to colleagues in these settings may form the beginning of vital partnerships. You may also consider networking with other colleagues who are interested in the use of self-management tools and perhaps share resources.

If you are interested in integrating self-help books or computer programs, consider working your way through the program one chapter or module at a time. This will help you decide if you think this book or program is appropriate for the patients you see. It will also provide you with first-hand insight into the challenges your patients face in completing self-help homework between sessions amidst other competing life demands. As with anything that requires an investment of time, it is essential to keep focus on the potential long-term return on your investment. In addition to potentially improving treatment outcomes, successful use of self-management may ultimately help you change your workload by shifting more of the responsibility for treatment to patients as active partners in self-management.

I am not comfortable changing the types of interventions I deliver

Ethical guidelines for mental health professions caution against practicing outside of one's area of expertise. In traditional professional training programs, clinicians gain specialization in a certain approach such as psychotherapy or psychopharmacology. Integrating other aspects of treatment such as meditation or exercise can begin to feel like you are stretching beyond your comfort zone. As such, it may be worth thinking about gaining specific expertise to build new competencies. For instance, obtaining training in the motivational interviewing techniques described earlier can help you become more effective at supporting patients in making lifestyle changes required for self-management. In terms of specific content areas, it may be worth considering attending a workshop on the application of meditation or exercise to the treatment of depression. Often such training may be offered in workshops that can be counted towards continuing-education requirements. The cost of such trainings may also be eligible for reimbursement if your workplace maintains funds for professional development.

I am not sure my patients will go along with this

You may wonder whether a particular patient would be willing to try self-management. Before asking about whether they would be willing to try a certain form of self-management, it may be especially helpful to ask each patient during the initial treatment planning phase about their past experience with different forms of self-management that you are open to integrating into a treatment plan. For instance, many patients will have used the Internet to look up information about depression. Many will also have had some period of time in their life when they exercised regularly. Self-help books are widely read and peer support groups are widely attended. Meditation is gaining increasing attention in mainstream media and is even offered in some schools and workplaces.

Asking patients about their past experience is an opportunity to discover clues about past success that can be built upon and challenges to be anticipated. If they have used one of these approaches in the past, what aspect was most helpful? What was most frustrating? If they have stopped using this form of self-management, why did this happen? Do they have any negative attitudes about this or other forms of self-management? As we discussed in the chapters on specific self-management approaches, it is crucial to correct misperceptions about the efficacy of self-management if prior experiences have been with unstructured or untested self-help approaches.

This discussion about the patient's past use of self-management and current preferences is an ideal way to contribute to the development of a collaborative approach to care. It is also crucial to convey to a patient the expected benefits of self-management, including a greater knowledge of factors that contribute to their depression and tools for managing it. Knowledge and skills can help to confer a greater sense of control over depression and a greater likelihood of staying well after they have recovered.

It is also helpful to keep in mind that each form of self-management may not be an ideal match for each patient's unique symptom presentation and situation. In each chapter, we provide suggestions regarding which patients may be better matches for certain approaches. However, rather than completely ruling out a given self-management strategy, it may be helpful to match interventions to a patient's current level of functioning. For instance, a patient with pronounced deficits in energy and motivation may have a greater likelihood of attending a peer support meeting than engaging in an exercise program, which may become more feasible as symptoms lift. Similarly, with certain interventions that require concentration, such as meditation, it may be helpful to have patients begin with brief daily practices of no more than 5 minutes. As concentration improves during the course of recovery, patients may be better able to engage with longer meditation practices.

I doubt my colleagues will go along with this

Some of the ideas we have presented can be implemented by a single clinician within the purview of treatment planning with their own clients. For instance, it is unlikely that a clinician would need approval from other colleagues in their practice to begin recommending that patients use self-help resources or attend a peer support group. Indeed, many surveys show that most clinicians already do this. However, suppose you think your practice could be improved through the hiring of a care manager, developing a web-based self-assessment program that is integrated with your clinic's electronic medical record system, or implementing a peer-led self-help program within your clinic. Such initiatives would likely require commitment of time and financial resources within the organization.

Indeed, some of the initiatives we have presented in this book would be challenging for even the most inspired clinician to single-handedly replicate in their own practice setting. Some of the research reviewed represents large undertakings made possible by infusion of grant funding or certain infrastructure resources available through the HMOs or socialized medicine settings in which the studies were conducted. In addition to resource and structural barriers, attitudinal barriers may exist among colleagues. As we have noted elsewhere, some components of self-management such as self-help and peer support may also be viewed skeptically by mental health professionals. We mention these obstacles to acknowledge that systemic changes in health care can require shifts in resources and attitudes. However, these challenges can be addressed.

If you feel passionately that some form of self-management would be valuable in your setting, there are several small steps you can take towards this goal. Before presenting your ideas about how self-management might be applied in your setting, it is wise to gather information that can strengthen your case. Such information gathering may also help you refine your original proposal. There are several types of information gathering that can be helpful both outside and within your practice setting.

First, it may help to read some of the original research studies reviewed in this book and listed in the reference section of each chapter. Reviewing these articles will provide quantitative data on the impact of self-management on clinical outcomes. Methods sections of studies often provide logistical details about how programs were implemented. Discussion sections often feature reflections on lessons learned and recommendations about how to optimize delivery of the self-management intervention. In short, take time to learn from the successes and setbacks of others who have introduced self-management in a treatment setting.

As a next step, informal discussions with colleagues can help you gauge their openness to integrating self-management. This may begin as a discussion of a particularly challenging patient with depression or a broader discussion of what barriers your colleagues encounter in treating depression effectively. Are there systemic changes that they think would be useful? From there, you may introduce the idea of self-management to gauge their willingness to integrate this into their practice. During the information gathering stage, it is important to listen carefully to their concerns and skepticism. There will be plenty of time to address unfounded skepticism and to help colleagues shift their thinking about self-management from a foreign concept to an opportunity, using some of the arguments presented in the chapters on self-help and peer-support. However, during this phase, it is important to remain open to ideas that might help self-management work optimally in your setting.

A third step may be to gather some preliminary data about the desirability and feasibility of a new program in your clinic. You may survey patients in your practice to gauge whether such a proposed change would be perceived as useful. As a next step, you may seek internal or external funding to conduct a pilot study to more systematically assess the desirability and feasibility of the program in your setting.

The more information you gather, the better prepared you will be to present your ideas to your colleagues and other stakeholders in your practice. Even if your presentation is persuasive, it is helpful to remember that change takes time. However, several trends are encouraging regarding the future of self-management. Research on self-management for depression is ongoing. New information technologies will increasingly make self-management more convenient and accessible outside of the clinic. We expect that HMOs will increasingly encourage patients to use symptom self-assessment tools as well as self-help and educational programs. We also expect that patients will increasingly expect a more collaborative and holistic approach to depression treatment. Given its promise, we believe that self-management will become increasingly integrated into treatment in both primary and mental health care settings. Time is on the side of self-management and of those clinicians eager to integrate it into the care they provide.

Index